age-less

wm

William Morrow
An Imprint of HarperCollins*Publishers*

age-less

THE DEFINITIVE GUIDE TO BOTOX, COLLAGEN, LASERS, PEELS, AND OTHER SOLUTIONS FOR FLAWLESS SKIN

FREDRIC BRANDT, M.D.,

WITH PATRICIA REYNOSO

HarperCollins books may be purchased for educational, business, or sales promotional use. For information please write: Special Markets Department, HarperCollins Publishers Inc., 10 East 53rd Street, New York, NY 10022.

FIRST EDITION

DESIGNED BY NICOLA FERGUSON

Printed on acid-free paper

Library of Congress Cataloging-in-Publication Data

Brandt, Fredric.
Age-less : the definitive guide to botox, collagen, lasers, peels,
and other solutions for flawless skin / Fredric Brandt with Patricia
Reynoso.—1st ed.
p. cm.
ISBN 0-06-051625-9 (hbk. : alk. paper)
1. Skin—Care and hygiene.   2. Beauty, Personal.   3. Botulinum toxin—
Therapeutic use.   4. Skin—Laser surgery.   5. Collagen—Therapeutic use.
6. Chemical peel.   I. Title: Ageless.   II. Reynoso, Patricia.   III. Title.
RL87 .B665 2002
646.7'26—dc21   2002026592

02 03 04 05 06 WBC/QW 10 9 8 7 6 5 4 3 2 1

CONTENTS

ACKNOWLEDGMENTS

Dr. Fredric Brandt would like to thank:
My patients, who through the years have inspired my creativity; my staff in Miami and New York; Patricia Reynoso, for adding style to my words; my personal assistant, Maggie, who is brilliant at keeping my life in order; my head nurse, Susie Salviejo; Dr. Andres Boker, research scientist extraordinaire; my agent, Lisa Queen, and my editor, Claire Wachtel, for their enormous patience; Nada Lantz at Lantz-a-Lot; Jacquie Tractenberg and Dana Tuchman at Tractenberg & Co.; Joy Behar; Bobbi Queen; our volunteers, Maija Arbolino, Brenda Segel, Linda Asch, and Andrea Cantor, who generously submitted their faces for everyone to see; our photographer, Sonja Pacho, and her talented team: Miok (hairstyling), Gail Goodman (makeup), Gina Appleby (styling), and Ronald Cadiz; my beautiful golden retriever, Sparky; and finally, the late Dr. Harvey Blank, former chairman of the department of dermatology at the University of Miami, whose vast knowledge continues to inspire me in the daily practice of dermatology.

Patricia Reynoso would like to thank:
Dr. Brandt, for always returning my phone calls; my husband, Euclide, for his endless reserves of patience and encouragement; my sister, for being my cheerleader; my friends and colleagues at W, Jane Larkworthy and Dahlia Devkota, for generously lending me out; and my twins, Brandon and Grace, whose flawless skin is so captivating.

FOREWORD

I have been a patient of Dr. Brandt's ever since he appeared as a guest on *The View* last year. We did a segment on collagen and Botox treatments, and I volunteered my face as part of the procedure. I will tell you that I was amazed and thrilled with his work, and I have been a devoted patient of his ever since. I never thought I would actually enjoy having needles put into my face! But every time I see Dr. B., I leave his office laughing and looking about ten years younger. Not a bad day!

I love the fact that I don't need to go under the knife and can leave his office and go about my business the same day. It's amazing how after only about a minute, I can see my lines looking softer and my entire face looking more youthful. I have told all my friends about Dr. Brandt's expert touch, and I completely trust his skill and judgment. The man is a magician. I'll be going to Dr. B. until I'm 103, or until the world runs out of collagen and Botox, whichever comes first. Bravo.

—JOY BEHAR

INTRODUCTION

I don't think I could have picked a more exciting time to be a cosmetic dermatologist. My twenty years in practice have exposed me to a multitude of patients seeking answers to the same burning question: how can we slow down this speeding train called the aging process? Clearly, there's no bringing that train to a halt—at least not in this era—but if there's one point that I try to convey to the men and women who sit in my chair it's that there's never been a better time to seek a little rejuvenation.

The last two decades have been incredible in terms of learning about what damages and prematurely ages the skin, and better yet, realizing how this damage can be prevented and even repaired. Before then, little was said about how aging is affected by sun exposure, smoking, pollution, deficient nutrition, and even stress. We thought lines and wrinkles were an unavoidable rite of passage and that a mediocre complexion could never be more than that. Persistent acne was tolerated, while sun spots were often blamed on eating too much liver. (I kid you not!) At best, a visit to the dermatologist was reserved for an itchy rash or a pesky wart. Finally, when it came to at-home skin care, most people reached for a bar of soap and perhaps slathered on cold cream if they were feeling adventurous.

Oh, how times have changed! Today we know that a suntan should come from a bottle of self-tanner and that your dermatologist's number is worthy of a spot on your speed-dial. Similarly, celebrating your God-given looks is admirable, but that doesn't make it wrong to want to improve on them. On a related note, our narrow definition of beauty has expanded enough so that finally, a Barbie doll's long, blond hair and blue eyes aren't the only standard to strive for. We've seen this in Hollywood, too. At this year's Academy Awards, Halle Berry, one of the winners, was just as breathtaking on the podium as Julia Roberts had been the year before.

One cannot discuss the effects of aging without bringing up the baby boomers. An estimated 76 million babies were born between 1946 and 1964 in the United States, forming a massive group of people who were prepared to fight their way into prolonged youthfulness. Today, the oldest baby boomers are entering their mid-fifties and the younger set are already in their late thirties. This means that we will probably see no end to this obsession with the aging process. Many of my patients are in this very age group, and if there's one sentiment that I hear over and over again, it's that while they understand they have to age, they plan to do it their way. Staying youthful and beautiful just for the sake of staying youthful and beautiful is no longer enough. Beauty equates with power and control, and for the baby boomers, that in itself is more valuable than anything else. To quote one of my good patients, "I thought I could age gracefully, but nah, that's out the window now!"

The influx of information and innovation that has hit the skin care market, both in products and in cosmetic procedures performed at a dermatologist's office, has had an immense impact on how we treat the aging process. The advent of "cosmeceuticals," an entirely new genre of skin care products that are known to deliver a biological action on the skin yet are sold over the counter, are a prime example of this. A host of ingredients are in this category; they include retinol, alpha and beta hydroxy acids, and antioxidants, with many others continually joining this prestigious group. Prescription skin medications, such as Retin-A, are also a great option for a significant number of people.

All this is reflected in the leaps and bounds happening in the dermatologist's office. It seems hard to imagine a time when a face-lift was considered the best solution for turning back the clock—a perception that couldn't have been farther from the truth, because when the face-lift was finally performed, the result was old skin that still looked old except it was now pulled back, not exactly the picture of youthfulness.

Plastic surgery remains a viable option for a lot of people, but it's definitely not the universal solution that it was once considered to be. We now know that a face-lift addresses only a portion of the aging process that is affecting your appearance. Issues like deep lines on the forehead and on the sides of the mouth, and skin that has lost its youthful glow, persist stubbornly even after the best surgery with the best plastic surgeon in town. The radiant fullness of the face is, in my opinion, one of the most important signs of youth, and plastic surgery will definitely not bring that back. Clearly, the key to erasing a few years from the face will not be found in the plastic surgeon's office.

This is the gap that superior at-home skin care and dermatological procedures like acid peels, filler injections, nonburning lasers, and Botox can fill. Together they allow you to control how you look, regardless of your chronological age. Bottom line: take care of your skin in small ways today, and you might not need to go under the knife tomorrow.

Even those who have already taken the leap into plastic surgery will benefit from taking charge of their skin. Whatever led them to the plastic surgeon in the first place will send them back there if they don't keep up the good work at home. I see many patients who have had facial plastic surgery, and I count them among my best clients. One female patient even told me that her hairstylist was accusing her of having had a second face-lift—he simply couldn't believe how rested and rejuvenated she seemed. When he demanded to know her secret, she told him that she'd been tinkering with Botox.

We cannot deny that attractiveness is still a very powerful tool. Like it or not, others judge us by our appearance. I'll even venture to say that there might never be a time when looks don't matter. But if there's one message I want to convey it's that beauty lies in the eye of the beholder—yours. Take advantage of the vast information and technology that you're lucky to have at your disposal and bring your very best face forward.

NOTE TO READER

This book is designed to provide information about the various remedies for aging that are presently available, to help you be a more informed consumer of these medical and health services. It is not intended to be complete or exhaustive; it is based solely on the professional opinions of Dr. Fredric Brandt, whose opinions may not reflect every physician's viewpoint. Before you undergo any cosmetic procedure, it is wise to have an in-depth consultation with your health care provider. The author and the publisher expressly disclaim responsibility for any adverse effects arising from the use or application of the information contained herein.

PART I

COVERING THE BASICS

one

: In the Beginning :

Riddle me this: What is the largest organ in the body? It regulates body temperature, protects us from dehydration and injury, and can have many sensations, including pain, heat, and cold? Need another clue? Its flawless, radiant appearance can make the difference between a good day and a fantastic day. Funny, isn't it, how the answer suddenly seems so clear.

The condition of the skin is a national obsession, and understandably so. Think back to the great beauties of our time (Grace Kelly, Marilyn Monroe, and Elizabeth Taylor spring to mind); and while they may have differed in coloring, hairstyles, physique, and fashion sense, they all had a common trait. You guessed it—they all possessed a complexion so awe-inspiring that the heart aches just looking at their photographs. We have our share of celebrated beauties today, and once again the common denominator is their smooth complexion, even skin tone, full lips, radiant glow, and utter lack of wrinkles. Beautiful skin is a valuable commodity and, better yet, one that is within reach.

Aiming for beautiful skin is a worthy goal, and we will be discussing the many ways to achieve it, but I also want to emphasize that just like any other organ in the body, the skin needs to be protected and cared for. When you tend to your skin—by shielding it from the sun's damaging rays, eating nutrient-rich foods, sleeping adequately, using superior skin care products, and entrusting its care to a dermatologist—it will reward you with an enviously healthy appearance.

Believe it or not, the skin has many other purposes besides its appearance. It:

- serves as an environmental barrier
- protects us from water loss and wounds
- has specialized pigment cells to protect us from the sun's rays
- helps regulate body temperature through the sweat glands
- involved in the production of vitamin D

: The Living Skin :

At first glance the skin seems pretty unremarkable, just a thin, flesh-toned covering for the body. But if you could peek inside, the sophisticated network within would amaze you. Generally speaking, the skin is divided into two layers: the epidermis and the dermis.

Epidermis

Whenever you study your skin or run your hands over it, you're touching the top layer, known as the epidermis. The epidermis partially is responsible for the skin's color, texture, and overall appearance. It also helps the skin stay moist by retaining water and acting as a barrier against the sun. Have you ever wondered how we're able to keep from getting water-logged in the rain, or when we swim? You can thank the epidermis, which is impermeable to water.

Topping the epidermis is the stratum corneum, and that is what we see when we're undergoing our weekly sessions with the magnifying mirror. This coating is made up of flattened epidermal cells, which lie on the surface of the skin in a basketweave pattern. These cells were once baby cells that, in a process called cell renewal, migrated to the top. In healthy adults, this process happens over a fifteen- to thirty-day period, but as we age, the process slows down considerably.

Further below in the epidermis are the three other layers: the transitional layer, the suprabasal layers, and the basal layer. In some ways, all are responsible for the overall health and beauty of the skin.

Dermis

In the world of beauty, the dermis is a virtual treasure trove, especially since it is where our precious collagen and elastin fibers reside. In fact, almost 70 percent of the dermis consists of collagen, with the remainder consisting of elastin, blood vessels, sebaceous glands, sweat glands, hair follicles, and immune system cells. This layer of skin is also incredibly resilient and can absorb a great amount of pressure.

But more important, let's discuss collagen and the role that it plays in the way your skin looks and behaves.

The Collagen Connection

When your collagen is plentiful and healthy, you will know it by what you see in the mirror. Think of collagen as your skin's mattress, and elastin as the coils that hold it together. Like everything else related to the aging process, our collagen is at its most abundant during the early childhood years; anyone who has admired a toddler's velvety skin can attest to that. Collagen production slows down in puberty, levels off in your twenties and thirties, and—you guessed it—grinds to a halt in your later years.

The beauty world is obsessed with keeping collagen safe and sound; and considering what a fundamental role it plays in beautiful skin, this fascination is totally warranted. Just as important, collagen helps to heal wounds and scars. Many creams claim to protect it, repair it, and regenerate it, but there is scant evidence that any of them actually follow through on these promises. (The only exception is the vitamin A derivative tretinoin, which studies have shown to have a positive effect on collagen.) Years ago, when antiaging skin care was in its infancy, there was an onslaught of "collagen" creams that claimed to boost natural collagen. Pretty soon, most people lost faith in them, realizing that the collagen molecule, which for those creams was derived from bovine, was too large to penetrate the skin's barrier. In other words, try, try again.

The fibroblast skin cells produce collagen, and it is the degeneration of collagen, through excessive exposure to the sun as well as extreme environmental conditions, that eventually leads to wrinkles and sagging skin. Once collagen is destroyed, it is very difficult to restore. Some of the latest non-surgical cosmetic procedures, like collagen injections and lasers, help repair the harm, but nothing will ever bring collagen back to its virgin state.

The Fatty Layer

Composed mostly of fat cells, the fatty layer lies beneath the dermis and works to insulate us and shield our inner organs from harm. This layer varies in thickness depending on where it is on our skin. Not surprisingly, it's pretty thick in the abdominal area, but almost nonexistent on the eyelids. Throughout the rest of the body, the fatty layer is also where cellulite, that universally dreaded condition, appears.

Elastin

Known as collagen's partner in crime, elastin is another connective tissue found in the dermis. These stretchy fibers allow the skin to snap back into place. Over time, and with repeated sun exposure, the elastin breaks into small fragments. There is no remedy for the destruction of elastin. When it's gone, it's pretty much gone.

: Our Skin Cells :

- *Keratinocytes:* The most abundant of all cells in the epidermis, keratinocytes provide some of the rigidity of the outer layers of skin.
- *Fibroblasts:* The kings of all cells, fibroblasts produce collagen.
- *Melanocytes:* Found in the epidermis, these cells produce the pigment melanin. As you're probably aware, melanin absorbs the harmful ultraviolet light produced by the sun and protects the skin's DNA from radiation damage. This pigment-producing cell also produces what is known as a tan—which sounds desirable until you realize that a tan is simply the body's response to injury from ultraviolet radiation.

FITZPATRICK SKIN TYPES

Developed by Professor Thomas Fitzpatrick, M.D., Ph.D., as a classification system based on skin pigment to calculate burning from sunlight, this system is commonly used to determine how the patient's skin reacts to the sun; it also serves as a guide for in-office procedures that will affect pigmentation.

Type I
Extremely fair skin, red or blond hair, blue or green eyes. Always burns, never tans

Type II
Fair skin, sandy to brown hair, green or brown eyes. Usually burns, difficult to tan

Type III
Medium skin, brown hair, brown eyes. Sometimes burns, often tans

Type IV
Olive skin, brown or black hair, dark brown or black eyes. Rarely burns, tans with ease

Type V
Dark brown skin, black hair, black eyes. Very rarely burns, tans very easily

Type VI
Black or dark brown skin and hair, black eyes. Never burns, tans very easily

- *Langerhans:* These cells are involved in the immune function of the skin.

: Skin Types :

It's impossible to approach a skin care counter intelligently without first understanding what type of skin you call your own. The typical classifications—oily, normal, combination, and dry—are still used today, but the rules for what constitutes what skin type aren't as hard and fast as they used to be. Most people may start out as one skin type and, as they age and their skin changes, wind up being something else entirely.

: In Harm's Way :

Considering how miraculous the skin is, it's shocking how easily we take it for granted and subject it to harm. Here, now, are the top five bad habits that stand between you and having the best skin you could possibly have. I'll be discussing these in more detail in Chapter 2: What Ages Us, but the topic is so important that I think it bears repeating.

1. Not using a sunblock: Keep this little formula in your head—You plus the sun minus the sunblock equals lots and lots of wrinkles.
2. Picking at your face: Have you ever taken a good look at what's lurking underneath your fingertips as you zoom in on your face? It's not pretty, and neither will your skin be, when it's left scarred and infected.
3. Not sleeping: Maybe it's the martyr in all of us that likes to brag about our amazing two hours of sleep, but do

this often enough and you'll be left with the skin to show for it. Take my advice and catch a few *zzzz*'s.

4. Stressing out: Our busy lifestyles have a way of turning us into hyperventilating manics, but before you continue to blow your cool, stop and remember that this is the easiest way to lower your immunity and affect the hormones that could cause your skin to flare up.

5. Inadequate nutrition: In the quest for a perfect physique, we have forgotten that starving ourselves can deplete our skin of essential nutrients. Trust me, a steady diet of rice cakes and diet soda will do nothing to enhance your complexion and lots to ruin it.

No matter what our desired end result, it's important to treat our skin respectfully and as best as we can. Believe me when I say that there's never been a better time to reach that goal. In the following chapter I will discuss the many transformations that the skin undergoes. Some, like natural aging, are going to happen no matter what our intentions, but a large part of them does lie within your control. Once you understand why your skin behaves and looks the way that it does, half the beauty battle is already won.

two

: What Ages Us :

When, exactly, did it all start? Where did our carefree youth disappear to, the time when only the occasional blemish could ruin our day? It's sneaky, I know, and even potentially distressing, but there's no way around the fact that aging will happen to each and every one of us. We might not be able to completely dodge the effects of aging, but understanding how and why it happens can teach us a lot about slowing the process down.

: Intrinsic and Extrinsic Aging :

There are two basic types of aging: intrinsic (or chronological) and extrinsic (or environmental). The first type, intrinsic aging, has to do with the inevitable passage of time and the conditions that arise because of it. In the 1960s, scientists discovered that the root cause of aging lay deep within our skin cells' DNA, which is why it's a good idea to glance at your parents to see what the future holds for you. Some of the conditions that come with intrinsic aging, which I will be describing in further detail later in this chapter, will happen no matter how well-intentioned you are. The good news—and anyone who is devoted to reading at least the occasional beauty magazine has certainly heard this before—is that there is plenty you can do to lessen their appearance. In fact, an entire industry is devoted to it!

The second type of aging is more sinister, if only because it falls within our control. Extrinsic aging is responsible for most of the harm that we view as aged skin, and it is brought on by external factors like smoking, pollution, sleep deprivation, poor nutrition, and of course the big one: exposure to the sun. Because this process is avoidable and usually self-inflicted, it is often referred to as premature aging. It's also important to note that skin cancer occurs almost exclusively in prematurely aged skin.

Intrinsic Aging—Signs Include:

- *Dry skin*: As we age, the skin's oil glands produce significantly less oil, resulting in pronounced dehydration that makes wrinkles more apparent.
- *Wrinkles*: The natural loss of those little worker bees, collagen and elastin, is largely to blame for the appearance of wrinkles. Years of dynamic expressions, in the form of smiling, laughing, frowning, and squinting, also contribute to wrinkles.
- *Large pores*: They're the bane of our existence, since they can make the complexion look rough and uneven. Some people are predisposed to enlarged pores (thanks, Mom!) while others are blessed with skin like glass. As we age, the loss of the skin's underlying support system prompts the pores to become even larger.

- *Redness*: A cluster of fine red lines appear most frequently on the cheeks and nose, and they're due to the proliferation of tiny broken capillaries underneath the skin.
- *Decreased healing capability*: Starting in our thirties, the turnover rate of epidermal cells slows down remarkably, resulting in both a dulled complexion and a decreased ability to heal wounds.

Extrinsic Aging—Signs Include:

In addition to the natural signs of aging, many people experience the following:

- *Increased roughness*: As free radicals, mainly from sunlight, destroy the skin's collagen and elastin, the skin cells start to turn over in an irregular fashion resulting in scaly patches of rough skin.
- *Spots everywhere*: Constant exposure to the sun's ultraviolet rays makes our skin pigment act abnormally, resulting in spots throughout the face, upper chest, and hands—basically, anywhere the sun has shone on.
- *Excessive wrinkling*: Even more pronounced wrinkling, particularly on the cheeks, neck, and forehead, is usually seen only in individuals who have been exposed to the sun.
- *Sagging skin*: Think of our elastin as rubber bands and the sun as a scissor. Now imagine that scissor (the sun) cutting the rubber band (elastin) into tiny pieces. How much bounce will those tiny rubber fragments now have? Not much, and that's exactly what happens with environmental damage.

ː So . . . What Ages Us? ː

As one birthday blends into the next, and the clock is ticktocking away, it's frighteningly easy to see how one can look up one day and realize, "Gee, I've aged." As we've seen, intrinsic aging is determined largely by your genetic predisposition. Truly, aside from asking for a different set of parents, there's little one can do to alter that aspect of aging. As for what constitutes extrinsic aging, the sun is a major contributor, but there are also others, like smoking, stress, sleep deprivation, and deficient nutrition.

The Sun

I like to think of myself as fairly easygoing—there's very little that irks me and much more that makes me laugh out loud. But if patients want to see me come undone, they'll visit me with suntanned skin. Actually, I should change that to the less seductive yet more realistic label "damaged" skin. On a daily basis I treat patients who are calmly waiting their turn at improving their complexions, yet they feign innocence when I ask about the telltale signs—usually dark spots coupled with bronzed, crinkled skin on their face, arms, hands, and most commonly their chest.

The excuses come fast. "I was wearing the sunblock that you gave me," swears the male half of the bronzed couple from Peru. Others are more belligerent: "I'm not going to stop living so that I can look good at eighty," says a thirty-two-year-old blond Realtor with a snazzy convertible and a love of boating.

Our dangerous love affair with the sun began almost sixty years ago. Before then, a tanned complexion was a sure sign that one labored outdoors for a living. Eventually, a tan became a badge of honor among the chic. It now signaled to the world that one had the means to spend weeks on a yacht on the Riviera. So pervasive was this image that even Coco Chanel fell under its spell, becoming the first designer to parade bronzed mannequins on the runway. If the message wasn't clear before, it certainly was now: being tanned was the ideal—at any cost. Just ask the Bain de Soleil model. Didn't she seem to be having a ball?

Appearances, no matter how utterly convincing, can be deceiving. The simple fact is that a darkened tone is the skin's immediate reaction to damage that has been inflicted on it. "Damage" is the operative word here, because it is this very damage that will, without a doubt, show up in your skin as premature aging. In other words, the majority of wrinkles and other signs of aging don't have to be there at all. For every cautious, sunblock-toting patient that I treat, I see five others flaunting their hard-earned tans, yet these are the same folks who will ask me to "do something" about the lines and spots on their faces and bodies.

This might be the twenty-first century, but perhaps a repeat lesson on what a tan really is is in order now.

THE FULL SUN STORY

Whenever unprotected (read: naked and devoid of sunblock) skin is exposed to the sun, an insidious cycle of damage is initiated almost immediately. The two ultraviolet rays that are found in sunlight, UVB and UVA, deliver their blows in different ways. The first, UVB, is often called the "burning" ray because of its power to do just that—burn. (Anyone who has ever dealt with a painful sunburn can thank good old UVB.) The other, the UVA ray, doesn't burn the skin; but because of its longer wavelength, it is able to reach deeper into the skin, down to the cellular level, where our DNA resides. Combined, the two activate the free-radical damage that we now know is largely to blame for the majority of skin aging, not to mention a host of other diseases, like skin cancer.

Living in Miami, the sunbathing capital of America, has provided me with ample examples, both in the office and outside it, of why we must limit the time we spend in the sun. Notice that I don't say "eliminate," because even I realize that people genuinely enjoy being in the sun. With that in mind, before dispensing advice about protection from the sun, I first try to ascertain my patients' lifestyle and the reasons why they're in the sun. If, for example, patients tell me that they love to golf, or that they regularly take their children to the playground, then we try to work around those outings. Believe it or not, staying away from the sun during the peak burning hours—11 A.M. to 4 P.M.—makes a significant difference in how much you damage your skin. I'm proud to say that I've been able to transform many of my patients with just this guideline. After all, life is too short to give up the things that truly fill us with joy.

This next piece of advice is almost simplistic, but since I am constantly given a multitude of excuses for being sunburned, I think it bears repeating. First, everyone needs to consider sunblock as vital as toothpaste and as indispensable as those pricey antiaging creams. No sunblock will offer you complete protection from the sun—you'd need to go outside covered with a metal cage to accomplish that—but the options today are so wonderfully diverse that it's truly inexcusable not to use one. In fact, the current crop of sunscreens is light-years ahead of its predecessors.

Until only a few years ago, traditional sunscreens only offered protection from UVB rays, partially because the non-burning UVA rays were, incorrectly, considered harmless. (Actually, one could get sunblocks that offered additional protection from UVA, but they were thick and opaque and very unpleasant to wear.) All that changed in the early 1990s when two major developments took place.

First, a process called micronization allowed makers of sunblocks to pulverize the traditionally thick, occlusive but very effective zinc oxide and titanium dioxide into fine particles that, when rubbed onto the skin, became nearly invisible. Finally, this allowed everyone, not just the lifeguards for whom this thick white stripe was a signature, to fully protect himself or herself from the sun in an appealing way. The other major turning point was the introduction of Parsol 1789, a chemical sunblock that is also known as avobenzone. (Until then, avobenzone was available only in Europe.) Avobenzone is an effective UVA blocker and it is now included in many sunblocks, in the process finally offering complete protection from both wavelengths of light. Today, pretty much every brand delivers this broad-spectrum protection.

THE LOWDOWN ON SPF

Unfortunately, the current system for calculating the sun protection factor (SPF) in sunscreens is far from perfect. It was originally developed to measure only the sun's burning properties. For example, if someone were to sit outside without any protection and become burned after a minute, a sunscreen with SPF 15 would allow him or her to stay in the sun for fifteen minutes before feeling burned. This calculation is effective for protecting against a burn, but as we now know, you don't have to get a burn to be damaged, since the UVA rays don't burn.

You might have noticed that SPF is available in a vast range of numbers, starting as low as 4 and climbing as high as 45. (Some European brands go as high as SPF 60.) Some sun protection is better than no sun protection, but in my professional opinion, you should stick to an SPF of 30, which is known to absorb 97 percent of the sun's rays.

In Europe, there is an entirely different system for measuring sun protection. In addition to measuring UVB, they also measure UVA radiation. If you pick up a European sunscreen, you might notice that in addition to SPF, printed on the bottle is an IPD number that stands for immediate pigment darkening. The higher the IPD number, the higher the protection against UVA radiation.

There's been a lot of controversy in the American market over how to measure the efficacy of sunscreens. Currently, when you buy an American sunblock, there is nothing that tells you how much UVA protection you are receiving; at present the only rating we have on our sunblocks are for the burning rays of the sun (UVB), not the complete spectrum. For now, look for sunblocks containing Parsol 1789, zinc oxide, and titanium dioxide.

The FDA plans to change the regulations for sun protection. The proposed change in the labeling system is that instead of SPF 30, the label could read SPF 30 Plus. The FDA system is notoriously slow, so I'm not holding my breath until any changes come. Until then, choose the best sunscreen available and practice reasonable avoidance of exposure to the sun.

DAILY DOSES

If you're anything like the majority of my patients, you're probably thinking that you can skip my lectures on the sun, since you're one of the smart ones; sunblock is the first item you pack when going on vacation or taking a long weekend away. While this sort of foresight is a step in the right direction, it falls short of the type of protection that is ideal. You see, the sun is out *all the time*, not just when you're on a beach in the Caribbean. It's out when you're driving to the office, running errands on a city sidewalk, or even dining indoors at your favorite restaurant. Yes, I said indoors—UVA rays are able to penetrate glass, so without adequate sun protection, you are at risk of getting some damage. Even in the dead of winter, you should make an effort to protect yourself. If not, over time this accumulated damage will greet you in the mirror: a leathery complexion, sun spots, and an abundance of lines, particularly the deep lines in a crosshatch pattern on the cheeks. Just think of the wrinkled neighbor in the movie *There's Something About Mary* to see exactly what you don't want to look like. Why wait until your skin is damaged beyond repair to start thinking about caring for it? Let's focus on preserving its beautiful integrity now.

CONCERNS ABOUT CANCER

On a more ominous note, research has shown that 40 percent to 50 percent of Americans who live to age sixty-five will have skin cancer at least once. Obviously, if you need another reason to avoid the sun, this is clearly the one.

DON'T LET THE SUN SHINE ON YOU

Once you've homed in on your sunblock of choice, you have to make a commitment to using it properly. Before you step outside, you should apply at least a teaspoon-sized portion to your bare face and give it time to be absorbed. Those with very sensitive skin should seek a chemical-free sunblock, such as one with zinc oxide or titanium dioxide; those with acne-prone skin should use a gel-based formula. Remember that sand and water reflect almost 100 percent of sunlight, so for that big outing on a bright day, make sure to have your new favorite product on hand and reapply it often. Finally, reach for a hat and sunglasses before heading outdoors. Just remember that a hat on its own offers almost negligible protection. A dark canvas hat that doesn't let any light show through is your best bet, although it does not protect against reflective rays.

A little-known but commonsense fact is that clothing offers a natural SPF. A white cotton T-shirt offers the equivalent of SPF 5 to 7, and switching to a black version ups the SPF to 20. There's even an innovative new product, Rit SunGuard, that allows you to add extra protection to your clothing simply by throwing it in the wash. The protectant that it contains ups the clothing's SPF to a minimum of 30 and lasts through almost 20 washes. Tinted windows, too, block UVA and UVB rays, as do the white gloves that many of my patients in Miami wear as they drive in the hot sun. (Those are my favorite patients!)

A new trend emerged a few years ago: makeup products, such as foundations, that came already loaded with sunscreen. While I think this is a step in the right direction, I still insist that you use a traditional sunscreen. Why? First, most of the new products feature only a minute amount of sunscreen. Second, and perhaps more important, recent studies show that sunscreen in makeup virtually disappears a mere two hours after application, leaving you with only the assumption of protection. Honestly, I resent the false sense of security that these products create. Bottom line: always use a separate sunscreen.

You've probably heard that we receive more than 80 percent of damage from the sun before the age of eighteen. Judging by the many patients who have sat in my office and reminisced about having suntanning competitions when they were teenagers, I'm not surprised. I think this fact is worth repeating, but I also hesitate to bring it up because some sun fanatics might interpret it as an invitation to indulge in even more damage. The damage is already done, right? But please, let's remember that those were the days when baby oil was the tanning tool of choice and ignorance was bliss; we now know that no excuse for voluntarily speeding the aging process is good enough. Even after years of tanning, someone who becomes serious about sun protection can achieve a great improvement in his or her skin. The body is amazingly efficient at fighting free-radical damage, especially when it's given a helping hand. I hope that the message is clear: embrace a natural aesthetic. Your face—and your dermatologist—will thank you for it.

Smoking

It's beyond me why anyone would still want to smoke after knowing how every single organ is affected by inhalation of the toxins involved. Perhaps I can appeal to your vanity by stating that smoking can also be destructive to your skin.

Formally, there are varying opinions about the effects of smoking on the skin. Some studies have found smoking doesn't harm the skin drastically, while others dispute such claims. My personal and professional opinion is that smoking adversely affects the skin in many ways. In fact, I can tell a smoker by his or her skin. Because smoking causes vasoconstriction, or decreased flow of oxygen and nutrients to facial tissue, smokers tend to develop a very sallow appearance. The skin tone is pale and a certain shade of gray. Smokers also get a lot more blackheads, because the pores are dilated owing to a decrease of collagen in the skin and they also don't heal as quickly as nonsmokers. This last point has even prompted many plastic surgeons to refuse to operate on smokers. At the very least, remember that smokers' lips are continuously pursed, causing lines on the upper and lower lip lines.

Deficient Nutrition

I believe strongly that if you take care of your body and your health, of course it's going to be reflected in your overall appearance. Vitamins and natural antioxidants found in food, such as the healing lycopene antioxidant that is so prevalent in tomatoes and green tea, to name just a few, help the skin stay healthy and functioning properly.

As a general guideline, eating fruits and vegetables, at least five servings daily, can be one of the best things you can do for your appearance. Foods like carrots and butternut squash contain beta-carotene, the precursor of vitamin A that keeps your skin—and your eyes—healthy. We know we live in a polluted world that increases the stress of oxidation in our bodies. Antioxidant-rich foods, like citrus fruits and broccoli, are great choices. Foods rich in vitamin E should definitely be part of your daily diet, as this antioxidant helps keep the skin healthy and vibrant. Look for vegetable oils, sunflower seeds, nuts, and seafood for your vitamin E fix. Water, at least eight 8-ounce glasses a day, is still a crucial aspect of keeping the skin hydrated and glowing.

It's important to also keep your body in good shape, as the natural consequence of too much fat, in the form of clogged arteries, won't allow enough blood to get where it needs to go.

Sleepless Nights

The next time you're tempted to trade a few hours of sleep for a few more hours at the office, remember that while you're snoozing, the body is recuperating. It is a known fact that while we sleep the body is working harder than ever to regenerate and unwind after the tensions of the day. While we sleep, our bodies are secreting growth hormones that are responsible for restoring cells and building skin, hair, and bone. Continue to rob your body of enough sleep and you'll start to see the consequences in your red, darkly circled eyes and dull skin. Do this often enough and it'll soon become clear how endless sleepless nights can add up to a less than beautiful reflection in the mirror.

Stress

A never-ending to-do list, a work schedule that just keeps getting more hectic, a boss who thinks that screaming is the best way to stimulate his employees . . . The list is seemingly endless and very few of us are fortunate enough to never feel its repercussions.

We know what causes stress, but what hasn't been emphasized nearly enough is what actually happens in a body under such duress. Cortisol is a hormone produced in the adrenal glands that is a key player in how well we handle stress. Cortisol serves a helpful purpose by providing us with that extra push to keep going, but when we force our bodies to overproduce it, that's when things can get hairy. Long-term exposure to cortisol can produce extensive damage to the body, including weight gain, and is considered a leading cause of premature aging.

Plus, all that scowling can lead to permanent wrinkling!

Pollution

Have you ever taken a walk down a congested city street during rush hour? If not, consider yourself blessed, since the fumes emanating from the bumper-to-bumper traffic alone are enough to make your skin cry out for help. Our often-mentioned ozone layer is at a scary all-time low, making us more susceptible to breakouts, irritation, and sensitivity. One study found that after prolonged exposure to ozone-depleted areas the skin's natural vitamin E content plunged by 25 percent. Similarly, dust can clog pores and increase the incidence of acne.

If a move to the countryside is not feasible, then try to limit the time you spend in heavily polluted areas.

When It Happens—A Decade-by-Decade Glance at Skin Aging

Thirties

In the third decade of life, we start to see the first signs that we have truly left our childhood years behind. That's when certain effects start showing up more, like puffiness under the eyes. Granted, some people have a genetic tendency toward puffiness, but more often than not, it's a sign of aging. Meanwhile, there might be some excess skin on the eyelid and the eyebrow starts to droop a bit. There might be a little fat accumulation in the neck, and the skin might lose a bit of its youthful radiance. Expression lines are just starting to appear around the eyes and mouth and in the forehead.

Luckily, you can slow it all down by protecting yourself from further bombardment by the sun. This is also a good time to incorporate an anti-aging product, like retinol, into your regime to boost your collagen reserves.

Forties

The picture starts to get more dire in the forties. Expect to see further loss of elasticity in the skin. A loss of collagen and fat will cause the cheeks to start heading south. The nasolabial folds—the smile lines—will also become more prominent. Any areas that experience a lot of movement, such as the eyes, will start to exhibit more wrinkling. The corners of the mouth will turn down, as if you were frowning. This is also when those annoying age spots start to deepen in color.

Decreasing levels of estrogen—estrogen dips before, during, and after menopause—are starting to make your skin drier than ever. On the upside, you might have less acne.

Fifties and Beyond

In the decade of the fifties, the changes that I've mentioned earlier become even more magnified. Again, loss of collagen and fat makes the face sag, and even the bony structure of the face starts to go. If you think of your skin as a sofa, the collagen within it can be compared to the cushy filling: as the filling decreases, the "sofa" deflates and sags. At this point, a face-lift would do a nice job of redraping all of this loose skin, but it can't replace the fullness that has been lost.

It might be disheartening to realize how everything seems to disintegrate as we age, but that shouldn't be how aging is perceived. The information that is available to us today is a valuable antiaging tool, allowing us to view the full picture and adjust accordingly.

It's been said enough to qualify as a cliché, but today, age truly is just a number. What that number actually looks like in the mirror is in your control.

three

: On the Home Front :

F ew can deny that regardless of your starting point, well-rounded, high-quality, consistent skin care is the most crucial factor in achieving and maintaining the skin of your dreams. Your genes might have predetermined your skin type, but this doesn't mean you have to live with skin that is less than flawless.

Admittedly, designing and ultimately sticking to the ideal skin care regimen is a pretty tall order. We live in a time when newness is valued above all else, relegating today's hot ingredient into tomorrow's old news, often long before you've had a chance to find out what all the fuss was about in the first place. Skin care has also changed dramatically: classics like cleansers and toners have been joined by a multitude of products that claim to exfoliate, purify, detoxify, lighten, and even amplify. Sometimes a single product professes to do all these things on its own! Factor in the countless brands of skin care products crowding department store shelves, each promising to be the latest and greatest innovation, and you can see how picking the right skin care products can become an exercise in utter frustration.

It doesn't have to be this way. Buying mounds of products that don't deliver on their promises doesn't have to be an accepted occurrence. Neither should perpetual confusion over what types of products will produce the best results for your specific skin type. The past twenty years have brought about significant advances in the skin care industry, and here's a news flash—a lot of them actually come through on their claims. Narrowing it all down is a matter of determining what actually works and what is just selling a pipe dream.

If I were to peek into my patients' medicine cabinets, I'm sure I'd be greeted with enough skin care products to moisturize a small foreign nation. Statistics reveal as much: a staggering $1.2 billion was spent solely on moisturizing products in the year 2000. Yet if the endless stream of questions thrown at me by my patients is any indication, a lot of women are still searching for the perfect product that truly works. While I don't think there is such a thing as a magic elixir—aging is inevitable, after all—I do believe that preventing flaws is far easier than fixing them. To that end, it's crucial to select skin care products according to basic criteria, such as seeking out ingredients that are proven to improve the skin, properly assessing the condition of your skin, and, most important, determining which goals are within reason. If you are in your thirties, for instance, maybe it's time to stop wishing for the skin of a teenager.

As a dermatologist, I have a lot of tools at my disposal to help the skin look its best, but contrary to popular opinion, I'm not a magician. Rather, I like to think of myself as my patients' partner, educating and guiding them toward an effective routine that will keep the skin as healthy and radiant as possible. We've come a long way in developing office techniques that can easily and dramatically rejuvenate the skin, but they are only half of the program. What a patient puts on her skin day in and day out is crucial—so much so that I can easily differentiate between my patients who are faithful to their cleansers, moisturizers, and eye creams and the rest who disregard my advice, usually on the assumption that I can easily fix everything. But honestly, what's the point of those pricey visits to the dermatologist and to your beloved facialist if you aren't maintaining all their hard work at home? I like to compare it to maintenance of the teeth: you continue to brush and floss long after a visit to the dentist, right? The same commitment should be devoted to your complexion.

In this chapter I will guide you through this dizzying maze of products and along the way, I hope, blast the perception that a skin care routine has to be complicated and time-consuming in order to make a difference in your skin's appearance. Also, at the end of this chapter, I will provide a guide to the many ingredients that I consider among the most innovative and effective.

: Treat What Ails You :

Problem: Hyperpigmentation

It's sometimes cute (a sprinkling of freckles across the nose) and sometimes not (dark spots on the chest and hands), but this much is true: hyperpigmentation is one of the most common complaints out there today.

Most pigment changes in the skin can be attributed to two major factors: hormonal shifts (pregnancy and the use of oral contraceptives are likely culprits) and prolonged exposure to the sun. An old injury, a disease, or an incorrectly administered cosmetic procedure can also contribute to this uneven accumulation of skin pigment in the form of postinflammatory hyperpigmentation. When the cause is hormonal, the pigmentation is called melasma, and it shows up as irregularly shaped blotches, usually on the cheeks, forehead, and upper lip. Melasma is a very common condition but, unfortunately, one of the most difficult to eliminate completely. A few lucky patients might see it go away on its own.

Solar lentigines, commonly known as sun spots, are a direct result of sun exposure and not, as many people believe, an unavoidable rite of passage. (Take a peek at an elderly person's naked body and you'll see that the vast spotting on the face and hands doesn't exist on the areas that have been protected from the sun.)

SOLUTION

Nearly every form of hyperpigmentation can benefit greatly from at-home bleaching products. Look for proven bleaching agents, such as hydroquinone. There are various other bleaching agents, such as kojic acid, licorice extract, and arbutin, which I will discuss later in this chapter. For hydroquinone, a standard concentration is 2 percent for an over-the-counter product and 4 percent for a prescription preparation. When these products are combined with retinoids and glycolic acid, which work largely by exfoliating the skin, penetration is improved and results are seen even faster.

Above all else, it's crucial that those with any type of hyperpigmentation become fanatical about avoiding the sun, since no other condition is as easily aggravated . Feeling an urge to step outside? Then by all means do so, but not without first loading up on a sunscreen that blocks both UVA and UVB ultraviolet rays of sunlight.

WHAT YOU CAN EXPECT

Given time to work, this regimen can significantly fade most signs of hyperpigmentation in one to three months, although those due to hormonal issues are usually more challenging to treat.

If there is a condition that lasers are superb at treating, it's certain types of hyperpigmentation. There is one caveat, however: only freckles and sun spots respond extremely well to laser treatment. (Conditions like melasma and other diffuse hyperpigmentation are more stubborn; for them, lasers are not the treatment of choice.) The lasers appropriate for hyperpigmentation are called pigment lasers and include the Q-switch ruby, Alexandrite, and Nd:Yag. Another effective solution is a superficial to medium-depth chemical peel, such as a trichloroacetic acid (TCA) peel. Both methods require several treatments before an improvement is seen. (All these in-office procedures will be discussed in detail in Chapter 6: Radiance Revealed.)

Problem: Acne

Everyone emits a huge sigh of relief when the teenage years are past, confident that the days of fighting acne are gone forever. I hate to burst this happy bubble, but I actually treat more acne in adults than in adolescents. Understandably, acne in adulthood is very distressing to patients, and they are often clueless as to how to rid themselves of it.

In adults, acne can often be traced to a mild hormonal imbalance, but there are other culprits, such as stress. Quite simply, acne results when the pore (technically known as a hair follicle) is blocked by dead skin cells that are never thoroughly expelled. Instead, the sloughed-off cells stick together inside the pore, and this plug, along with the accompanying sebum, then becomes a source of nutrition for bacteria. The bacteria then greedily invade the pore and cause redness and inflammation. In all, not a pretty picture.

As acne heals, it might sometimes leave the complexion with a dark spot. Those plagued with this condition often refer to the spot as an acne scar, but that's actually incorrect. Rather, it's an inflammatory response to acne that leaves behind a change in the pigment in the skin. By comparison, a scar leaves a textural change in the skin. In any case, it may take a few months for these spots to go away, but their appearance is helped greatly by a light peel or a prescription vitamin A product.

SOLUTION

Now for the good news: with the many acne treatments that are available today, adult acne can soon be as distant a memory as your yearbook picture. Topping the list of highly effective antiacne ingredients are retinoids, which are derivatives of vitamin A that work by controlling the cell stickiness that is the primary cause of acne. The most popular retinoid is tretinoin, and it can be found in the prescription medications Retin-A, Retin-A Micro and Avita, both of which are FDA-approved for the treatment of acne. Other retinoids are tazarotene (found in the prescription medication Tazorac), adapalene (Differin), and to a slightly lesser degree retinol, which is found in many products sold over the counter. Certain oral contraceptives, such as Ortho Tri-Cyclen, have FDA approval for the treatment of acne and are helpful for those patients whose acne is a result of mild hormonal imbalances.

Significant improvement can be obtained by unclogging the pore. Salicylic acid, a beta hydroxy acid that is lipid-soluble and can therefore penetrate the sebaceous material in the follicle, is simply magical at this. Salicylic acid is found in a multitude of products, even cleansers. Finally, it's very helpful to use a topical antibiotic, such as clindamycin, to control bacteria. Benzoyl peroxide is not only another reminder that your teenage years will live on forever; it's also a very effective, commonly used antibacterial ingredient in many over-the-counter acne medicines. Many of today's acne preparations contain up to 10 percent benzoyl peroxide, which is a pretty significant amount. Its only downside is that it may provoke an allergic reaction in a small group of people. Finally for acne that is very resistant to other topical treatments, there is Acutane. However, this is an extremely potent oral medication that requires an in-depth discussion with your doctor.

Supplement It With

An in-office salicylic acid "beta" peel, usually at 20 percent to 30 percent, administered every couple of weeks, is an excellent partner to an acne-fighting home routine. Glycolic peels can be used to treat acne, but I prefer salicylic acid peels for the same reasons that I like salicylic acid in general. Its unique fat-soluble composition permits salicylic acid to penetrate deep into the pore and clean it out thoroughly.

What You Can Expect

As long as the patient is committed to a maintenance program, acne is a very treatable condition. But patience, at least eight weeks' worth, is crucial, since the skin needs time to regenerate.

Problem: From Fine Lines to Furrows

Ah, wrinkles. They seem to be the symbol for aging, and they are the focus of nearly every slick advertisement for skin care flashing across your television screen. A preoccupation with all types of lines and wrinkles is likely to start in a woman's late twenties to early thirties, when she sees the first indication that she's no longer a teenager. In younger women, the presence of wrinkles is usually linked to a premature degeneration of collagen and elastin from sun damage. In time, however, everyone, including people who were diligent about sun protection, will end up with some wrinkles. Wrinkling is inevitable, but there are ways to slow down its progress.

SOLUTION

Because this problem has many reasons for being, the solution is just as multifaceted. First and foremost, reduce the risk of accumulating further wrinkles by staying out of the sun. Next, one of the easiest approaches to reducing wrinkles is to keep the skin amply moisturized, since any type of dryness may exaggerate them, particularly around the delicate eye area. Last, start incorporating products with retinoids, which are proven to increase collagen, in turn alleviating wrinkling. Your dermatologist can guide you toward the right formula for your specific level of wrinkling. It's also a good idea to supplement your skin care regimen with products rich in antioxidants, such as green tea and grapeseed extract, which protect the skin from further damage.

WHAT YOU CAN EXPECT

Once a wrinkle has made itself comfortable on your skin, it's nearly impossible to remove altogether with topical treatments. (Hence, my motto Prevention Is Everything.) But if you become vigilant about avoiding sun damage and stick to a consistent skin care routine, you can expect those pesky critters to become softer and more diffused.

Almost every in-office cosmetic procedure is aimed at reducing the appearance of all types of wrinkles. People with only minor lines can start small (a light acid peel or a series of microdermabrasion treatments), while more serious cases can benefit from any number of procedures known to stimulate collagen, such as lasers and deeper peels.

Problem: Sensitive and Irritated Skin

Sometimes, identifying your specific skin condition can turn into a guessing game in which you never seem to have the answer. One of the best examples of mistaken identity is skin that is irritated and overly sensitive. Since redness and peeling, usually around the nose and forehead, are characteristic of sensitive and irritated skin, the problem is often dismissed as just "dry skin." In some cases, the patient may be genetically predisposed to this type of skin, which may become easily irritated when the patient is under stress. A polluted environment, especially in large cities, can also make the skin overly sensitive, as can harsh skin care products.

Solution

In dealing with sensitive and irritated skin, the logical first step is to calm it down, either with a soap containing zinc or with a low-dose hydrocortisone cream. Natural, plant-based ingredients like rosemary and aloe are also fantastic at soothing the skin. A standard regimen might involve using a combination of such ingredients for approximately a month. After the skin has settled down, it can probably tolerate more active ingredients that in the past weren't a viable option for such sensitive skin.

The peeling, rough texture will be vastly improved and the uncomfortable tightness alleviated.

Problem: Uneven Texture and Loss of Radiance

Often, what stands between "good" skin and "flawless" skin can be seen right on the surface. A complexion that is uneven and dull can be attributed to a number of culprits, but the most common is a decreased rate of cell turnover, often brought about by sun damage and aging. Any behavior that interferes with the microcirculation of the blood, such as smoking, can also be blamed for a dull cast on the skin.

SOLUTION

Babies' skin is often synonymous with a smooth, velvety finish. While we might never get back to that point, it is entirely possible to take a few steps back. First, analyze why the skin is uneven and rough to the touch. In most cases, the culprit is an accumulation of dead skin cells that haven't been properly removed. In these instances, the key word is "exfoliation." Look for products containing alpha and beta hydroxy acids— that is, glycolic and salicylic acids. Depending on how much your skin can tolerate, you can devise a complete program around these active ingredients. Many of today's cleansers feature these acids, but if you have to choose just one method for getting your acid fix, you should find a product that will remain in contact with your skin. And remember that all retinoids work by unmasking your youthful glow. When dullness is a result of hyperpigmentation, a bleaching product would be a great addition. If it's because of smoking . . . well, you know what I'm likely to say about that.

As with everything else related to skin, patience is the word of the day. Dull, lifeless skin didn't happen overnight, so you can't expect it to improve overnight. The good news is that after at least a month on a steady, glow-inducing regimen, you can expect to have substantially smoother, more radiant skin.

HOW TO IMPROVE YOUR SKIN IN . . .

One Week

The clock is ticking, but don't despair; there's plenty that you can do in just seven days to make over your skin. When time is of the essence, exfoliating the skin offers the fastest route to improvement. For this, you will need the bare essentials: a mild granular scrub, a pore-cleansing clay mask, and anything with glycolic and salicylic acids, which get the job done like nothing else. A possible regimen can consist of a mask every other night, with the scrub on alternate nights. Both treatments will help to remove superficial buildup. The salicylic acid product will clean the pores even further, and glycolic acid will remove any stubborn residue. If necessary, finish with a coat of moisturizer.

One Month

The previous combination of salicylic and glycolic acids, mask, and scrub offers you a great head start, and you can now supplement it with a vitamin A product such as retinol. Experiment with different versions and concentrations until you find one that your skin can tolerate. I guarantee that it will be worth the effort, since nothing improves the condition of your pores and gives the skin such a beautiful clarity as this ingredient. Finally, prevent any barely visible brown spots from becoming darker by adding a bleaching ingredient like hydroquinone.

: The Bottom Line :

All your most burning questions about skin care—answered.

Are Facials a Necessity or a Huge Waste of Time?

Unlike our European counterparts, we are not a nation that values pampering rituals like facials. Usually, as the aesthetician is busy slathering our faces with multiple potions and lotions, we're busy thinking there must be something more productive that we should be doing instead. The many new day spas that opened in the mid-1990s increased the interest in facials, adding a sense of urgency and obligation to facials as a crucial step in a skin care routine. There are many benefits to having regular facials. The pores get professionally cleansed, the facial massage stimulates the skin's microcirculation, and the concentrated percentages of active ingredients that are applied are a rare treat. And, of course, anything that makes you feel this relaxed is going to have a positive effect on your skin.

If facials make you feel great, then by all means indulge. Just remember that a facial is a supplementary treatment, not a replacement for a consistent home care routine. Your facialist may truly be amazing, but the benefits received from one treatment will not carry you until your next appointment unless you do your share at home.

What Is a "Clinical Result," and Why Should I Care?

As a physician, I'm trained to cast a critical eye on all types of statistics and supposed success rates that don't have broad, solid research behind them. In particular, I'm referring to those glossy television commercials and magazine ads for the latest antiaging discovery that flaunt many impressive-sounding test results. These results may indeed be reported accurately, but the circumstances behind the testing are never fully revealed— and they are a factor that could paint a totally different picture. For example, how many participants were in the study, and just how bad was their skin to begin with? Also, remember that the companies themselves sponsor these studies, so they can't be expected to be 100 percent objective.

I'm not implying that every marketing campaign behind an antiaging product is full of hot air. Simply, don't blindly believe everything that you hear just because it's in an enticing commercial with a gorgeous twenty-year-old model.

Is a $300 Cream Worth Every Cent?

What is it about creams with astronomical prices that makes perfectly sane women, and a handful of men, too, run to the stores to stock up on them? Judging from my patients' mixed testimonials, a lot of this hype might be a tad undeserved. That pricey miracle cream may have made your best friend's skin glow, but this doesn't mean it will do the same for you. I realize that there's something very exciting about buying a luxurious cream with the price tag to match, but any informed consumer will see past the glamour.

But, to be fair, it is sometimes necessary to place a higher price on certain creams simply because higher-quality ingredients are more expensive. Some of the drugstore lines, for example, can't make use of certain raw ingredients because it would simply cost too much, a cost that they would have to pass along to their customers.

Does Anything Truly Help Collagen Production?

The master of all selling points in beauty advertising has to be the one that promises increased collagen production.

Considering the critical role collagen plays in the beauty and health of the skin, it's not difficult to understand why. Years ago, when the antiaging revolution was just beginning, the most popular creams were collagen-based. The premise was that since collagen is so crucial to flawless skin, a cream with collagen in it would replenish the skin's natural supply. Before long, women realized that their skin didn't look all that different. A little softer, perhaps, but those lines were still hanging on for dear life. Why? Quite simply, the collagen molecule is too large to penetrate the skin when applied topically. (This is why collagen is usually injected into the skin.) It's not going to be of much benefit if it can't make its way inside!

Today, the only ingredient proven to stimulate collagen production is retinoid, famously found in Retin-A and Renova, among others. The scientific data on retinoids have proved that these derivatives of vitamin A can penetrate deep into the skin's dermal layer, where the collagen resides. Other studies have also demonstrated, albeit less definitively, that vitamin C may also increase collagen synthesis.

Are These Pores Mine Forever?

They're as annoying as mosquitoes on a balmy summer night, but unfortunately, the 20,000 pores that are spread out across your face, particularly the large pores that often make the skin look rough and uneven, can't simply be swatted away. There are several reasons why the pores have this unattractive appearance. It is true that those with oily skin tend to have larger pores than those with normal to dry skin, but this is just a guideline, not a hard-and-fast rule.

The biggest reason is that as we age and lose collagen, this decreased elasticity results in the enlargement of the pores. I always explain it to my patients in this way: Think of a straw (the pore) floating upright in Jell-O (the skin). As the Jell-O starts to melt, the straw loses its balance. In this analogy, it makes sense that stimulating the collagen in the skin can result in firmer skin and a smaller pore.

Contrary to what you might have heard, it is impossible to change the size of your pores permanently, since pore size is determined by genetics and age. Keeping the pores clean, with professional facials and a combination of alpha hydroxy and glycolic acid, can help make them less prominent. Finally, don't underestimate the power of a little makeup!

: Routine Matters :

The bare essentials of at-home skin care.

Cleanliness Counts

Today's cleansers are a sophisticated bunch, as they not only remove the day's grime but can also provide tangible, long-lasting benefits. This wasn't always the case. There was a time when the only option for cleansing the facial skin was a bar of soap, and anyone who's suffered from terribly dry skin can attest to how harsh soaps are. I like to tell my patients to save the deodorant soap for when they're truly filthy, and even then use it only on the body. Moisturizing bars came next, and they were a big improvement over traditional soap, as they cleansed without stripping the skin. The best-known moisturizing bar is Dove, and I still recommend it to my patients who like the feel of a bar.

Many people like liquid cleansers, and—given their ease of use and versatility—it's easy to see why. Unbelievably, liquid cleansers have been around only since the mid-1990s. It was then that the technology was invented, allowing for a wider choice of ingredients in a significantly milder formula.

As for what type of cleanser you should choose, this depends on a number of factors. Someone with acne-prone skin, for example, might do well with an exfoliating cleanser containing glycolic or salicylic acid. Even though a cleanser remains in contact with the skin for barely a minute, in that short time it will have prepped the skin to receive an exfoliating cream and better penetration of the cream will be achieved simply because of the cleanser. Similarly, botanicals such as green tea are extremely soothing, and a cleanser that is chock-full of such ingredients is beneficial for those with sensitive skin.

As a general rule, those with dry skin should opt for a creamy cleanser that has very little foaming action, oily skin does well with foaming gel cleansers, and those lucky enough to have normal skin can use pretty much anything. Cleansing twice a day is ideal, but if you absolutely cannot clean more than once daily, I recommend doing it at night. It's been said a million times, but going to sleep with a face full of makeup is an open invitation to breakouts and dull skin.

These days, it's hard to walk down a skin care aisle without seeing those handy facial cleansing wipes. If the convenience of a wipe that's pretreated with cleanser appeals to you, and might even make you more conscientious about cleansing, then hooray for technology.

Tone

There's something about toners that people love. Toners are actually relics of the days when most cleansers left a heavy residue on the skin and one needed to remove it by taking this extra step. Today's cleansers pretty much clean up after themselves, so a toner with strong astringent action is unnecessary, in some cases, not to mention dehydrating. A benefit is derived, however, from using a toner that is formulated with active ingredients, such as those with antioxidants and gly-colic or salicylic acid. If you choose to use such a toner for these benefits, just keep in mind that the percentage of active ingredients in a toner isn't as high as what you'd find in a cream.

Moisturize

There's something comforting about a moisturizer, if only because it's such a traditional part of the skin grooming pro-cess. Nearly every complexion can benefit from a mosturizer, even an oilier one.

Moisturizers don't take years off your age, but they perform another function that is almost as important: they keep your skin hydrated. And as anyone who has experienced the tight-ness and itchiness of dehydrated skin can attest, hydrated skin is comfortable skin. Also, a good moisturizer helps minimize the appearance of fine lines and wrinkles, and this is perhaps just as important.

As the uppermost level of the skin, the stratum corneum, confronts a daily assault from the environment, a moisturizer works by creating a barrier between it and the air. Without this barrier, the skin would flake and become irritated. Another important feature of a moisturizer is its ability to help the skin maintain its own water reserves.

A good moisturizer usually contains both occlusive ingre-dients (to prevent loss of water) and humectant ingredients (to attract water from the atmosphere and from the deeper layers of the skin). In the first category, common occlusive ingredients are petrolatum—yes, as in good old Vaseline—and mineral oil. Other occlusive ingredients that are very effective at retarding water loss, as well as imparting a smooth texture to skin care products, are grapeseed oil, squalene (from olives), soybean oil, beeswax, paraffin, dimethicone (a type of silicone), and lanolin. As useful as these ingredients are, however, they are effective only while on the skin; once they are removed, the skin's natural water-loss function returns to normal.

Humectants, meanwhile, are able to attract water from the atmosphere and from deep within the skin itself, causing a slight swelling of the uppermost skin layer that gives the appearance of smoother skin with fewer wrinkles. Commonly used humectants include glycerin and some alpha hydroxy acids, particularly lactic acid, hyaluronic acid, sorbitol, propylene glycol, urea, and sodium lactate.

Most, but not all, facial moisturizers also include emollients. These substances, which include dimethicone and propylene glycol, are added to help soften and smooth the skin and function by filling the spaces between the skin cells to create a smooth surface. Actually, many emollients function as humectants and occlusive moisturizers as well. An emollient is a very helpful ingredient in a moisturizer, as it's been shown that a well-hydrated stratum corneum makes the skin more stable and less vulnerable to irritants.

Of course, many of today's popular moisturizers, whether oil-based or water-based, don't just hydrate. (And besides, where's the sex appeal in that?) A moisturizer containing antioxidants, such as vitamin C and green tea, performs a double duty by adding an extra source of protection.

Protect

Without a doubt, positively and absolutely, there is no product more important to the health and beauty of your skin than a sunblock. If I had my way, I'd get rid of the sun altogether—that's how detrimental it is. But in the real world, a sunblock is the second-best choice, and it should be considered as essential as your toothpaste and toothbrush. Several studies have been done on identical twins who have led different lifestyles, and in case after case it was found that the twin who diligently protected her skin had far less damage than her reckless (or perhaps just uninformed) sibling.

An easy way to incorporate sun protection into your lifestyle is to use moisturizers with a built-in sun protection factor (SPF). Or, simply find a sunblock that suits your skin type and use that as your moisturizer instead, every day, prior to heading outside. Trust me, not only is it extremely easy to incorporate into your routine, but it will save your skin.

(For more on the role of the sun in aging, please refer to Chapter 2: What Ages Us.)

Extra, Extra

EXFOLIATION

Sometimes, even a sophisticated organ like the skin needs a bit of assistance in performing what should come naturally. Exfoliation, the loosening of dead skin cells from the upper layer of the skin, has risen in prominence, and with good reason. That accumulated debris dulls the complexion, more so as we age and our cell turnover slows down. Regular use of an exfoliant, either in a scrub or in an exfoliating agent like glycolic and salicylic acid, helps the skin along. It also allows better penetration of the moisturizer that follows it.

But it is easy to become overzealous about exfoliating. If a granular scrub is your preferred tool, choose one with perfectly spherical particles, such as jojoba beads, that don't scratch the skin. Also, don't rub too vigorously. When it comes to exfoliating, it is possible to have too much of a good thing.

Surely you've been lectured about how the eye area is the most delicate on the face and should be carefully tended to. But if you're like many harried patients that I treat, an eye cream is likely to be the thing you abandon. This is a big, big mistake.

The eye area suffers from a lot of cosmetic problems. It gets wrinkled easily, and it might have some crepiness and a proliferation of visible blood vessels that show up as darkness under the eyes. It might also be more sensitive than the rest of the face and become easily irritated. And since it has few oil glands, it becomes easily dehydrated.

For all these reasons, an eye cream is an absolute essential. Look for formulas with the most potent moisturizing and wrinkle-fighting ingredients. Even better would be one with a built-in sunscreen for an extra dose of protection. If you're truly lacking the time or the inclination, then go ahead and use your regular moisturizer in this area. Hey, even I do that sometimes.

Routine Odds and Ends

Orderly Fashion

First you cleanse, then you tone—you'd be surprised at how many people still get that wrong!

But seriously, the order of products is determined by how many, and what types, of products, your routine consists of. For example, I often advise my patients to use a vitamin A product, like prescription retinoids or over-the-counter retinols, only at night. These powerful ingredients tend to make the skin extra-sensitive to light and can leave your skin terribly burned if it's not properly protected. Also, the sun can decrease the ingredient's efficacy.

Protective antioxidants, such as green tea and grapeseed extracts and vitamin C, are ideal for daytime use. If a bleaching product is a part of your routine, you can safely add it on top. Top it all off with a moisturizer, if necessary.

If your routine incorporates several active ingredients, it's best not to use them simultaneously. Some brands of skin care products brag about having a combination of active ingredients like glycolic and salicylic acids in the same bottle. The assumption is the more, the merrier. This, however, isn't a beneficial feature, since most acids tend to work more efficiently at different concentrations and pH levels and their combination in a single product might cause them to inactivate each other.

PATIENCE, PATIENCE, PATIENCE . . .

At the start of any new skin care regimen, the prospect of flawless skin can make us giddy with excitement. As days go by and that dream skin has yet to make an appearance, it's easy to become discouraged and fling the products into the trash, only to start all over again with a new assortment of products. This is all understandable—and I've seen it dozens of times with my patients—but trust me when I say that it'll all pay off in the end.

New products, particularly those with collagen-stimulating properties, need ample time to work; there's no way that this can be accomplished overnight. I advise my patients to try out their new products for at least a month (two or three months would actually be ideal, but I know how impatient we can all be) before moving on to the next thing. The fact is that you aren't going to see any improvement in your skin after just a few days. One exception is an exfoliating product, which tends to remove surface dullness quickly, leaving you satisfied that you're making progress.

BEAUTY FIRST-AID KIT

Sometimes, despite doing all the right things to keep your complexion flawless, a disaster will happen at the most inopportune time. You can ensure that intruders like puffy eyes, dull skin, and blemishes disappear as quickly as they arrive by keeping your "beauty first-aid kit" fully stocked. The following five ingredients are all you need:

1. green tea bags

2. brown sugar

3. milk

4. ice

5. clay mask

Depuff your eyes: Moisten green tea bags with water and chill them in the refrigerator for a few minutes. Lie down with the chilled bags over your eyes. The polyphenols in the green tea are an anti-inflammatory agent, and the cooling reduces swelling.

Instant radiance: Grind brown sugar with warm milk and let the mixture cool to room temperature. This is a great scrub, since it exfoliates in two ways: the lactic acid in the milk acts as a mild exfoliant, and the sugar granules deliver a scrubbing action.

Deflate a pimple: When a blemish is really red and inflamed, an ice cube placed over it will instantly calm it down. Follow that with a dab of a clay mask to dry out the pimple.

: The Skin Care Library of Ingredients :

Cosmeceuticals

The term "cosmeceutical" was coined by the famous dermatologist Albert Kligman, M.D. Without a doubt, the advent of skin care products featuring these cosmeceutical ingredients—

from retinol and alpha hydroxy acids to vitamin C—has revolutionized the way skin behaves and looks.

In 1938 Congress passed a statute known as the Federal Food, Drug, and Cosmetic Act that set up the criteria for what a drug is and isn't. Traditionally, a drug has been defined as a substance that can treat and prevent disease, or bring about a change in the body. On the opposite end of the spectrum are cosmetics, which are classified as inert substances that only cleanse or enhance the skin's appearance. Cosmeceuticals fall somewhere between, since although their manufacturers claim that they may cause a significant and tangible change in the skin, they are easily found in beauty and department stores, and no prescription is necessary.

A lot of what's competing for your attention at beauty counters actually works; but that said, the extensive benefits that these products promise should still be taken with a grain of salt. As a dermatologist, I am trained to cast a questioning eye at antiaging products that have scant proof for what they're claiming, and I advise my patients to try to do the same. Perhaps this isn't always the fair approach, but it's far too easy for people to be fooled by a glamorous marketing campaign.

For now, with the exception of retinoids, no claims about a products' antiaging effects have been evaluated by the FDA and given its official stamp of approval. To get such an approval requires a process that is comparable to sending a few rookie astronauts to the moon; it's so exhausting and costly that most skin care companies decide to soften their claims and do without this endorsement.

Now that you know what a cosmeceutical is, let's talk about what a cosmeceutical *does*. And that, in one word, is plenty. Pretty much everyone can derive benefit from a cosmeceutical product. Actually, you might have already indulged and never even realized it. Here, now, are a few cosmeceutical superstars proven to deliver many benefits, from smoothing lines and wrinkles to restoring the radiant glow of your youth.

Vitamin A

RETINOIDS

If you're starting not to love your reflection in the mirror, then a vitamin A product is one of the best investments you could make for yourself. Years of scientific research have proved that certain vitamin A derivatives, typically categorized as retinoids, can significantly improve years of accumulated sun damage, clear up acne, and—since they increase collagen synthesis—even help with chronological (non sun-induced) aging. In fact, tretinoin, as found in the prescription medication Retin-A, was originally approved by the FDA for the treatment of acne. It turned out to be more versatile than was originally thought, as patients on Retin-A were soon reporting that their skin felt smoother and less wrinkled after treatment. After numerous studies came to the conclusion that tretinoin did indeed help with wrinkling, the same active ingredient was then approved for the treatment of fine wrinkles associated with chronic sun exposure and natural aging. Its name was Renova, and it remains the only product proven to help with wrinkling.

Some irritation, in the form of redness and flakiness, is normal when tretinoin is first used. It's a good idea to start by applying it every other night until the skin gets used to it. No matter how much I tell my patients that these irksome side effects are quite normal, and a sign that the active ingredient is actually doing something, many still become discouraged and stop the treatment. If this has been your experience, I would suggest that you either alter how often you apply it or try a different concentration. You can expect to see a reduction in fine lines and wrinkles in approximately three months.

Years after retinoids, in the form of Retin-A, first hit the market, scientists went back to their laboratories to uncover a version that could be available over the counter. The result was retinol, a close relation to tretinoin that must first be converted to retinaldehyde and then to all-trans retinoic acid in the skin. In other words, it's a step away from the more active tretinoin, but also less irritating and nonetheless very effective. Many studies have shown that retinol can significantly improve skin texture and clarity, sallowness, mottled hyperpigmentation, pore size, fine wrinkling, and overall photodamage. It's also very effective at increasing the moisture content in the skin. This was an amazing discovery, especially since it would now be available to a larger group of people; but as often happens in the highly competitive world of skin care, many products claiming to contain retinol don't work as well as they should. Why? In order to deliver such benefits, retinol

Over the last several years, those mad research scientists have been working diligently to modify the original molecular composition of retinoids, in the process creating many types (or generations) of retinoids. All possess—to varying degrees—the ability to reverse the signs of aging; and with the exception of retinol, all are available only by prescription.

- Tretinoin (found in Retin-A, Retin-A Micro, Renova; and Avita)

- Retinol

- Isotretinoin

- Adapalene (found in Differin)

- Tazarotene (found in Tazorac)

must be manufactured, formulated, and packaged properly to avoid loss of potency. Also, the concentration of active retinol must be high enough, usually 0.04 percent to 0.07 percent, to make a real difference in the skin. Telling you that a lot of skin care companies take shortcuts is like telling a child that Santa Claus doesn't exist, but I'm doing it simply to make you aware that not all skin care products are created equal.

The Acids

If you're one of those people who cringe at the thought of applying an "acid" to your face, then you're truly doing your appearance a disservice. This family of naturally occurring acids, headed by alpha hydroxy (AHA) and beta hydroxy (BHA) acids, have the ability to exfoliate and smooth the stratum corneum and speed the cell cycle (which is slowed in aged skin) like little else out there today. Some evidence even suggests that AHAs, primarily glycolic acid, can stimulate collagen production.

There was wide acceptance of acids when they were first introduced in the early 1990s, perhaps because many people soon discovered how quickly these ingredients worked. Many others, however, complained of irritation and prematurely decided that the entire category of acids was inappropriate for them. Because there are hundreds of AHA products available today, the category can be both confusing and misleading (not all work the same way). But this also means that there's an acid out there for everyone.

Now, meet the family.

ALPHA HYDROXY ACID (AHA)

Anyone who has contemplated using an AHA product has probably been overwhelmed by the vast assortment of products with this ingredient. Granted, there are many types of

AHAs, and they all work to varying degrees, but what unites them, aside from their similar molecular structure, is that all are derived from natural sources. These sources include sugarcane (glycolic), sour milk (lactic), citrus fruits (citric), apples (malic), grapes (tartaric), and rice (phytic).

Of this group, you've probably heard most about glycolic acid; this is because, quite simply, glycolic is the most effective at improving the overall appearance of the skin. This benefit is largely due to its small molecular size, which makes it able to penetrate deepest into the skin. Every benefit seems to have a downside, and glycolic is no exception, since it is also the most irritating of the AHAs. As with retinol products, not all AHA products are interchangeable. Unlike retinol, however, AHAs are not unstable, so proper packaging is not as crucial.

What is so crucial to getting great results is the concentration of the active ingredient in the product. Not surprisingly, not all AHA products contain a high enough percentage to actually change the skin. Typically, most AHA creams have 4 percent to 8 percent of active AHA—enough to give a slight zest to the skin but not nearly enough to deliver that "wow" factor. To make matters even more confusing, the vast majority of AHA products don't list the percentage on the package. Why? Because the FDA has said that they don't have to. Also, even if you found an AHA cream with a fairly high percentage, that still wouldn't paint the entire picture, as the pH level is of major importance. The pH level is the level of acidity; the lower the pH, the more acidic the product. Naturally, the more acidic the product, the better it works, but it then has a greater potential of causing irritation.

BETA HYDROXY ACID (BHA)

Who knew that a powerful skin care ingredient resided deep in the heart of willow bark and sweet birch trees? I'm referring to salicylic acid—a beta hydroxy acid (BHA) and a key ingredient for restoring clarity to the skin. Salicylic acid has an anti-inflammatory effect, making it very useful for patients with acne and rosacea. This acid also has a distinct advantage over glycolic: because it's lipid-soluble, salicylic acid is able to penetrate the oily material blocking pores, in the process exfoliating and cleaning them out. It is also slightly milder than glycolic.

POLY HYDROXY ACID (PHA)

In the quest for an active ingredient that would be minimally irritating and could therefore be tolerated by many, a new category of hydroxy acid has been created: poly hydroxy acid. Early studies are finding that PHAs are indeed very gentle, but that they do not work either as quickly or as efficiently as AHAs or BHAs.

Why should you use an acid? Here are five great reasons:

1. It smooths the top layer of skin without disrupting the skin's barrier function.
2. It may boost collagen production, in turn reducing wrinkles.
3. Some acids, like salicylic acid, are able to enter and exfoliate the pores.
4. Some acids, like lactic acid, are fantastic moisturizers.
5. An acid helps fade hyperpigmentation.

Botanical Garden

They have a long tradition, but botanical ingredients—such as those from plants, flowers, and herbs—are the most modern way to get a beautiful complexion. The way I see it, who can argue with the ancient civilizations that relied on aromatic substances for many purposes, including fragrances, cosmetics, medicine, and cooking? I personally like them for their proven healing, hydrating, and antiseptic properties, which carry over extremely well into skin care. Also, when combined with active dermatological ingredients, botanicals can help take some of the sting away.

Here are a few of my favorite botanical ingredients. They are all widely used.

ALOE VERA

It's been said that Cleopatra attributed her beauty to aloe vera gel, and today aloe vera is a popular base ingredient in many skin care products. Aloe is a healing emollient that works wonders for the complexion, soothes irritations, and prevents scarring. It is also used to reduce swelling associated with arthritis, and it has been effective when eaten to control blood sugar. Finally, aloe also regenerates injured nerves and is excellent for soothing rashes and burns.

CHAMOMILE

You've enjoyed it piping hot in tea, yet chamomile has many other uses. Egyptians dedicated this plant to the sun, and in sixteenth-century Rome it was used for its anti-inflammatory and soothing action. Today, its power to soothe and reduce irritations associated with blemished skin makes it an important ingredient in skin care products.

GRAPESEED OIL AND EXTRACT

The use of grapes in cosmetics dates back to the seventeenth century, when, at the court of Louis XIV, it was fashionable to apply mature wine to the face for a radiant complexion. The skin-lightening action of grapes was also well known to French vintners. It is now known that the grape juice extract used in cosmetics is rich in a variety of sugars and contains a significant quantity of tannins, vitamins, and fruit acids, which have softening, whitening, and protective effects. Grape-seed extract is a powerful antioxidant known to fight free radicals; it is also known for its pharmacological ability to protect collagen, elastin, and essential tissue elements in the skin.

LAVENDER

Originally used to relieve muscle spasms, nervousness, and headaches, lavender has been noted for its curing effect against bacterial infections and flu viruses in its oil form. As a topical ingredient it acts as a soothing and calming element for both the skin and the senses.

LICORICE

Cultivated for medicinal purposes, the root of licorice is harvested after three years in the ground. Licorice has been used since the Middle Ages, and it has been used in Chinese medicine for its anti-inflammatory and antibacterial properties, and is useful in treating skin ailments such as eczema and psoriasis.

WITCH HAZEL

Witch hazel was named by Indian tribes because of its resemblance to the hazel tree. The leaves have become a classic treatment for troubles affecting veins; they are known to strengthen the resistance of the small blood vessels that can often burst under the skin. In some skin care products, witch hazel is used for its refreshing sensation and astringency.

Avocado

The avocado tree grows in tropical regions. It was introduced to Europe during the Middle Ages, and its delicious fruit was highly sought after. The flesh of the fruit is used to calm, soothe, nourish, soften, and hydrate the skin.

Rice Bran Oil

An ingredient considered magical in Asia, rice bran oil has been found to reduce cholesterol and lower the risk of cancer when taken internally. Topically, it has an impressive ability to impart a healthy glow to the skin and shine to the hair.

Tea Tree Oil

Long regarded as a useful topical antiseptic agent in Australia, tea tree oil (*Melaleuca alternifolia*) has a variety of antimicrobial qualities. It has been shown to work as well as benzoyl peroxide on acne. True, it takes longer to work, but it doesn't have as many side effects. Tea tree oil is also known to relieve pain and has an antipus action when applied to the skin.

Rosemary

Its Latin name is *rosmarinus*, "dew of the sea"—where it loves to grow. Rosemary increases circulation and acts as a tonic, which can be effective for treating combination and oily skin.

Shea Butter

Native to Africa, the shea tree bears wonderful fruits and grows in the savanna. An African legend says that these trees are the "wefts of our lives' dreams." The butter itself is obtained from

the shea nuts. Not only does it leave the skin with a soft and
and silky texture; it has a powerful antioxidant action.

MATÉ

Also known as yerba maté, this widely cultivated evergreen
tree is indigenous to Paraguay, Brazil, and other parts of South
America. The leaves are used medicinally as a diuretic, tonic,
and central nervous system stimulant and to relieve fatigue.
Maté has a high antioxidant value linked to the rapid absorption rate of phytochemicals found in its leaves. Finally, it is
known to stimulate the immune system.

GUARANA

The first recorded use of guarana dates back to 1669, when the
Maue Indians used it as a daily tonic and stimulant. It contains tetramethylxanthine, a compound almost identical to
caffeine. The fact that the seed is fatty means that absorption
is time-released into the body and skin. Overall, this ingredient has an energizing effect on the skin.

KOLA

In traditional African folk medicine kola is used to cure stomach ulcers, diarrhea, dysentery, and other ills. Muslims consider kola nuts sacred. In skin care products, kola acts as a
stimulant to assist in the action of other ingredients and their
absorption into the skin.

GERANIUM

The most widely used types of geranium come from both a
British and an American plant. In skin care products, the

antiseptic qualities of geranium make it helpful in treating acne, bruises, broken capillaries, burns, and eczema.

SOY

In Asia, soy has been known for centuries for its health benefits. In Southeast Asia, where soy protein is consumed by more than half the population, there are lower rates of heart disease, osteoporosis, and many cancers. In skin care, it's a fairly new ingredient that is very nourishing and healing.

SUNFLOWER

The sunflower is a tall plant whose large heads of yellow flowers follow the sun all day as it moves across the sky. Its name is derived from Greek mythology. The North American Indians praised the medicinal and nutritional virtues of sunflower and revered it as a divine plant that resembled the sun. Sunflower seeds yield an oil that is used for cosmetic purposes because of its moisturizing and protective properties.

Antioxidants

As we go about our daily lives, our bodies are continuously assaulted by a variety of harmful free-radical molecules. It's a process that medical professionals have differing opinions on, but this much is true: these free radicals are to blame for the vast majority of skin aging.

Here's how it works: A free radical is an oxygen molecule that has somehow lost its partnering electron and is now crazily searching to fix the situation. The way it does this is by latching onto healthy skin cells. Once a healthy skin cell has been altered, it too is now an unstable, unhealthy cell and eventually affects the way the skin cells multiply and turn over. The body naturally produce free radicals, since they're a by-product of natural activities like breathing and digestion. However, the major factors in damage by free radicals are environmental conditions like sunlight, cigarette smoke, and pollution.

The body is a miraculous instrument, and it has the ability to repair this damage by using a host of its own healing components, called antioxidants. The body's defense mechanisms include hundreds of antioxidants. The five that are most commonly used in skin care products are vitamins C and E, glutathione, lipoic acid, and coenzyme Q10. This particular group of antioxidants is called "network" antioxidants, as they have a fascinating ability to help one another regenerate. This is necessary because after an antioxidant has disarmed a free radical, it is no longer able to function unless it is recycled. Just like a bunch of army buddies, these antioxidants help each other return to their antioxidant state.

This natural system is amazing, but a daily lifestyle that includes far too much time basking in the sun defeats our ability to defend ourselves. When our protective system is compromised in this way, the body is said to be in a state of oxidative stress and cannot, on its own, fend off the potential damage. Steps in the right direction include boosting our diet with antioxidant-rich foods, avoiding the damage in the first place, and, naturally, using a skin care product rich in numerous antioxidants.

In this section I will be reviewing some proven antioxidants: green tea extract, which is just starting to emerge as a superstar antioxidant, grapeseed extract, vitamin C, and vitamin E.

Green Tea Extract

From my point of view, it's pretty hard to dispute the many impressive findings that are being revealed about benefits associated with green tea.

Green tea is proving to be as potent on the skin as it is inside the body. The data released on the powers of green tea were just too impressive to ignore. I was already a believer, and that is why I had already incorporated such a high amount into my skin care products; but after reading about the latest data, I decided to boost the levels of green tea even further.

A lot of the medical studies that have been released on green tea found that when it is applied on the skin it protects the skin from ultraviolet light and may even help prevent skin cancer. Daily oral intake of green tea helps prevent prostate cancer. The studies have been so positive and convincing that I feel strongly about sharing them with you here.

The Green Tea Story

Americans might be devoted to their morning coffee, but for many Asian cultures, drinking tea is just as important. Except, of course, that the custom of drinking tea is actually doing the body a great service.

The Japanese custom of drinking green tea came from China about A.D. 800, and it started when Buddhist monks, who had gone to China to study, discovered how healing green tea was. Upon returning to Japan, the monks brought the tea back as a medicinal beverage.

For centuries, green tea has been lauded for its healing properties. In the Kamakura era (1191–1333), the monk Eisai wrote a book *Maintaining Health by Drinking Tea* (1211). In it, he wrote: "Tea is a miraculous medicine for the maintenance of health. Tea has an extraordinary power to prolong life. Anywhere a person cultivates tea, long life will follow. In ancient and modern times, tea is the elixir that creates the mountain-dwelling immortal."

Clearly, green tea has from early times been highly valued as a powerful medication. But in recent years research into the effects of green tea has progressed so far that it can now provide scientific confirmation for what was believed at that time.

Strongest of All Antioxidants
Found in Green Tea . . .

In September 1997 a study by Dr. Lester Mitscher, a professor of medicinal chemistry at the University of Kansas, concluded that green tea contains the strongest of any known form of antioxidants. The study found that a cathechin in green tea, epigallocathechin gallate (EGCG), was more than a hundred times as effective at neutralizing free radicals as vitamin C, and twenty-five times more powerful than vitamin E. Both are well-known antioxidants. (As I mentioned earlier, antioxidants are thought to prevent cellular damage that leads to certain diseases—especially cancer.)

Mitscher indicated that green tea contained, by far, the highest concentrations of active EGCG. He also stated that the daily amount of green tea needed for an antioxidant effect had not been established, but he cited previous studies in China and Japan, where people customarily drink four (or more) cups per day. It has not been determined whether one cup per day is sufficient.

Green Tea as a Cancer Preventive

Continuing research on the benefits of green tea for human health has produced several new findings. Most notable is a study by Japanese scientists of the Saitama Cancer Research Institute relating the delay of cancer onset with the consumption of green tea. The study shows that early-stage breast cancer spreads less rapidly in women with a history of drinking five or more cups of green tea a day. As a result, there is a lower recurrence rate and a longer disease-free period.

With the evidence that green tea and EGCG, a catechin found only in green tea, are natural and readily available inhibitors of a gene expression which promotes the growth in cancer cells and in their surrounding tissue, it is possible for researchers to extend this idea to other various human diseases. Since EGCG has also been found to kill cultured cancer cells without causing harm to surrounding healthy cells, green tea could be beneficial not only in preventing cancer but also in preventing and treating other diseases.

Medical Studies

In a series of tests conducted on mice, the mice were first inoculated with cancer cells and then studied for the growth of malignancies. One group was given an extract of green tea; a control group was not given this extract. Comparison of the two groups showed a marked reduction in the growth of tumors among the mice receiving green tea. In further joint research with Professor Shu-Jun Cheng of the Cancer Institute, Chinese Academy of Medical Science (Beijing), mice were given substances which, when transformed in the body to cancer-causing chemicals, generate carcinoma in both the esophagus and stomach. The researchers then proceeded to check if green tea had the ability to inhibit the development of these cancers. Administration of green tea extract did indeed reduce the incidence of cancer to less than 50 percent. In addition, research at the National Cancer Institute (Tsukiji, Tokyo) found that administration of catechin (the main component of green tea tannin) to mice previously given chemicals that induce duodenal cancer can also significantly lower the incidence of cancer. Green tea and its component catechin have, therefore, been found to reduce the growth as well as the actual generation of cancer.

We do not yet fully understand the mechanism underlying

the generation of cancer, but according to one theory it involves at least two stages. A substance capable of causing mutations (initiator) first damages DNA in the cell and renders it subject to cancer (initiation). This condition then remains unchanged for some time until another substance, which activates cancer (promoter), leading to the actual growth of a malignancy (promotion). It is clear from recent research that extract of green tea and catechin can markedly inhibit both stages of development.

Even though these results have been gained from animal studies or pure laboratory tests, I think it highly possible that green tea and its component catechin have the ability to prevent cancer in humans.

Other benefits of green tea as an oral antioxidant:
- Restricts the increase of blood cholesterol
- Controls high blood pressure
- Lowers blood sugar
- Suppresses aging
- Deters food poisoning
- Fights viruses

Drinking Green Tea Reduces the Effects of Smoking Cigarettes

The effects of green tea on oxidative stress, brought on by the toxins of cigarette smoke, were investigated in two studies, one by scientists at the Academy of Preventive Medicine in Beijing, China, and the other by James Klaunig at the Indiana University School of Medicine in Indianapolis. Oxidative stress appears to cause or participate in the development of certain diseases, most notably cancer.

Researchers found that when cigarette smokers drank an equivalent of six cups of green tea a day, they suffered 40 percent to 50 percent less oxidative damage to their bodies than people who smoked the same amount but didn't drink green tea. This potentially lowers their risk of cancer, emphysema, heart disease, and other illnesses. However, it is important to note that those who drink green tea and continue to smoke are still raising their risk of oxidative damage. Nonsmokers who drank green tea exhibited significant decreases in oxidative damage as well.

So . . . How Does Green Tea Work on the Skin?

Free radicals, known to cause four out of every five wrinkles in the skin, have surely met their nemesis in green tea. Green tea on the surface of the skin works to prevent aging, owing to its extraordinary ability to protect essential tissue elements and antioxidant reserves in the skin. Medical studies have found that when green tea was painted on one arm and not the other, after thirty minutes of UV exposure the arm with green tea, when analyzed on a cellular level, did not suffer the changes induced by UV radiation in the unpainted arm.

GRAPESEED EXTRACT

Often touted as having more antioxidant powers than both vitamin C and vitamin E, grapeseed polyphenols are known to increase the strength of the blood vessels and protect collagen and elastin fibers.

VITAMIN C

Famous for its instability, vitamin C remains a potent antioxidant. The version featured in most products is ascorbic acid, which is also found in human skin. Ultraviolet radiation lowers the skin's ascorbic acid reserve, compromising the amounts needed for collagen production. A lot of after-sun skin care products contain vitamin C, as it is known to prevent prolonged harm from free radicals.

VITAMIN E

Topical application of vitamin E may reduce adverse responses to the sun, such as redness and swelling. Many people who have heard of this vitamin's wound-healing abilities break open vitamin E capsules and rub the liquid onto their skin. This can actually be very irritating; however, there's no disputing that this antioxidant is essential for our general health and beauty. Vitamin E is found in many vegetables, seeds, and nuts.

Whiteners

While Americans are entranced by sun-kissed skin and will actually harm their skin to obtain that glow, women in Japan are obsessed with the very opposite idea. For centuries, the Japanese ideal has been a porcelain complexion, with not even a hint of a spot to be found anywhere. Remaining speck-free surely takes some planning and care, but Japanese women get a lot of help from a skin care ritual that has existed in their culture for years: bleaching creams, also known as whitening or lightening creams.

Unless you've been parked under a parasol all of your life, you're probably well aware of these spots and want to get rid of them—now. This is where skin whiteners come in. First, I must set the record straight. If you use a whitener and your skin is naturally dark, your skin will remain exactly the same color; you will not be following Michael Jackson's lead in becoming part of an entirely different race. That said, it's important to note that a whitening cream works on the affected areas by retarding or blocking the production of melanin. The ingredients work slowly, so again, patience is called for. Also, using it with tretinoin, glycolic acid, or other whitening ingredients maximizes the effect. Now that we're clear about this, read on. The most commonly used whitening ingredients are:

- Hydroquinone—Controversial enough to be banned in Europe and highly regulated in Asia, the chemical hydroquinone is still the most widely used and most effective whitening agent. It is also FDA-approved for this use, but in low concentrations, usually 2 percent for over-the-counter preparations and 4 percent in prescription formulas.
- Arbutin—Traditionally used in Japan, arbutin is found in the leaves of pear trees and certain herbs. For those who are reluctant to try hydroquinone, arbutin is a suitable substitute, but it may not deliver the same results.
- Kojic acid—Widely used as a food additive, kojic acid is also valued for its stability.
- Others—Mulberry, licorice, and thyme extracts; azelaic acid.

New Names on the Block

Our country is built on innovation, and the skin care industry definitely shares this trait, as it is always madly searching for the latest and greatest antiaging discovery. A definitive guide on skin care wouldn't live up to its title without a look at newfangled ingredients that have gotten a lot of media buzz. In my professional opinion, these ingredients are worth noting because the manufacturers are making pretty big claims, but since no long-term studies have been performed yet, I would recommend that consumers don't dip into their wallets without first knowing the whole story.

COPPER

Copper is the third most abundant trace metal in our bodies (after iron and zinc) and it is present in virtually every one of our cells. (Interestingly enough, the American diet features less than a milligram of copper a day.)

Copper's chief responsibility is to activate the antioxidant enzyme superoxide dismutase, which in turn helps the body fight off free-radical damage. In 1996, the first FDA-approved gel for wound healing featured copper as its primary ingredient. It was able to penetrate the skin, thanks to its delivery system, the peptide complex. Other proven uses of copper have been in areas of hair loss and in soothing the skin after procedures like laser resurfacing, dermabrasion, and chemical peels.

Recently, talk has revolved around copper's ability to help repair photoaged skin. One study found that copper peptide was more effective than other ingredients, including vitamin C, in stimulating collagen production. Not surprisingly, there are now two major copper antiaging creams on the market, one available only in high-end department stores and the other in drugstores.

KINETIN

If kinetin, which is a growth factor, can keep green, leafy plants living longer, imagine what it can do for human skin—or so goes the thinking behind this ingredient. Whether this is really the case has not been answered very definitively. The makers of creams featuring kinetin claim that it may be as efficacious at improving the effects of photoaging as retinoids, without the problem of causing sensitivity. One study concluded that kinetin, like copper, spurs production of an important antioxidant. Another study, this one performed at the

University of California, Irvine, reported significant improvement in fine wrinkles, mottled hyperpigmentation, and rough skin. Kinetin is also said to help the skin retain its moisture for longer periods of time. As impressive as these early findings are, there isn't long-term proof that kinetin truly does what it is said to do. For me, more studies are needed before I can truly get excited over kinetin's possibilities.

Until very recently, creams featuring kinetin were available only at a dermatologist's office. Today, an entire range of kinetin products can be found at your local drugstore, both in the skin care aisle and in the cosmetics aisle. Yes, that's right. The same maker is featuring kinetin in makeup, including lipstick. Whoever said fighting off the aging process was too time-consuming? Just swipe and go!

Is your mind spinning? Admittedly, this is a lot of information to digest, but I hope I've provided you with a solid foundation to help you build an effective—and enjoyable—skin care program.

PART II

BEAUTY OPTIONS
AND TECHNIQUES

magine building your dream home with nary a tool in sight. No hammer, no drill, no power saw—kind of difficult, isn't it? Now apply this same logic to the mission of staying youthful-looking for as long as possible. Should you be expected to sit back and simply hope for the best? Of course not, and with the best of today's nonsurgical cosmetic procedures, you certainly don't have to.

An understanding of the elements that constitute an aged appearance, in combination with access to the best procedures for doing something about those elements, is a winning combination. For years, conversations about aging revolved solely around those dreaded lines and wrinkles: how to prevent them, how to erase them, and eventually how to live with them. The problem with this simplistic approach to aging was that it didn't focus on the other elements, which had little to do with a few crow's feet around the eyes. We now realize that many characteristics describe a youthful face, including a full face and lips, elevated eyebrows, and a firm neckline. Unfortunately, as we age, most of these features slowly start to go the way of the high school prom.

: Our Antiaging Toolbox :

Today, we understand that treating the effects of aging goes far beyond just treating wrinkles. As a cosmetic dermatologist in the bustling cities of Miami and New York, I treat male and female patients who bombard me with mile-long lists of their concerns about beauty. I like to tell them that my work is not just about filling and erasing lines; it's also about bringing back an overall youthful appearance to the face. This entails analyzing the patient and determining which elements are contributing to making him or her look tired and not as fresh. Often, wrinkles are a major factor, but they are not the only factor. Sunken cheeks, dark circles under the eyes, and facial features that seem to be heading south are equally guilty, as is the loss of facial fat.

Here's where advances in nonsurgical cosmetic treatments come into play. Often referred to as "lunchtime" procedures, these options include everything from Botox, collagen, fat, and silicone injections to microdermabrasion. Some, like chemical peels and collagen injections, are certainly not new, but their use continues to be refined and they are still ranked among the top five cosmetic procedures, as of last year. (These figures are courtesy of the American Society for Aesthetic Plastic Surgery, and they're based on a range of all cosmetic procedures, including surgical procedures like face-lifts and nose reshaping.)

The advent of Botox as a bona fide rejuvenating treatment has been a long time coming, and if there are any naysayers left, they surely can't argue with the FDA's recent approval of Botox for the treatment of frown lines. Botox is one of the most versatile procedures available today, and it has fulfilled people's demand for instant gratification. I liken it to digital pictures or even the Polaroid camera—we want great results and we want them this instant. This injectable has made people realize that there's no need to wait until their looks fall apart before dabbling in cosmetic procedures. A few shots of Botox erase years from the face and—just as important— refresh the complexion and impart a serene glow.

Collagen injections, meanwhile, are hanging tight, although the competition is certainly nipping at their heels. The biggest news in filler materials, which work by adding flattering volume to the face and softening wrinkles, are the hyaluronic acid fillers. The most popular version is Restylane, and I personally think that once it's formally approved by the FDA, it will revolutionize the industry just as Botox did. With Restylane, I am able to restore natural volume to the face and fill in lines and wrinkles instantly. The best part is that we can do this without a need for a skin test, and the effects last for a long time.

: Why Are the Procedures Appealing? :

Why have millions of men and women signed up for these procedures? The answer is actually quite simple: the procedures work! I've learned that people want the most impact with the least possible commitment of time. They also want little to no recovery time, low risk of side effects, minimal discomfort, and, ultimately, striking results. I think it's safe to say that these procedures deliver all this.

Another major factor in choosing these temporary procedures has to do with people's apprehension over plastic surgery. I often have patients tell me that after weighing their options, they've chosen to undergo a few less invasive procedures. Their reasons vary. Often, they're afraid that they might look radically different, they're turned off by a lengthy recuperation period, they've seen one too many "bad" face-lifts, or quite simply they might not need plastic surgery yet. But I like to stress that if you're not at the point of having surgery, this doesn't mean you shouldn't try to maintain your looks. These procedures are ideal for tinkering with various aspects of aging without drastically changing your overall appearance.

Also, contrary to popular opinion, plastic surgery

does not cure all ills related to appearance. A face-lift, for example, is great for lifting sagging skin and for tightening the neck, but it will do absolutely nothing for lines, wrinkles, and imperfect skin.

: Who Are These People? :

It's easy to imagine that only the most photographed and wealthiest people in the world have these procedures, but on the basis of my practices and my long career as a cosmetic dermatologist I can testify that this is absolutely not the case. For every celebrated person whose looks are directly tied to popularity (and paychecks!), I also get a so-called ordinary patient. "Ordinary" patients run the gamut from schoolteachers to lawyers to businessmen and businesswomen to stay-at-home moms. Their reasons for dabbling in cosmetic procedures that slow down the aging process are just as diverse. Some want to preserve their looks, while others feel that being rejuvenated and staying attractive will help them remain competitive in their chosen fields. One of my good patients in Miami, a woman in her mid-forties, has recently returned to college; her Botox injections make her look as refreshed as her classmates who are more than twenty years younger.

The last chapter in this book will bring to life just how rejuvenating these procedures can be. Four women whose ages range from almost forty to the mid-fifties, with different concerns about beauty, have been rejuvenated with a mix of Botox, collagen, and Restylane.

These three procedures were chosen because they deliver the most impact with the least investment of time. I invite you to see for yourself just how rejuvenating a visit to the dermatologist's office can be.

: One-Stop Shopping :

The great advantage of these procedures is that they can be combined for an even more dramatic effect. One unbeatable combination is Botox, usually for eliminating crow's feet and lifting the brows, and a filler like Restylane wherever a little extra volume is needed and on deeper wrinkles that need softening. Every so often I'll see a new patient who comes in with a predetermined idea of what procedure she'd like to have and is delighted to hear that conditions she considered untreatable can also be treated on the very same day.

: Top Ten Questions to Ask a Doctor :

You've done the research, your best friends are smugly flaunting their flawless new complexions, and, yes, you've grimaced one too many times in the mirror. Clearly, it's time to undergo a little cosmetic rejuvenation of your own.

But where do you go? It's one thing to make the decision to indulge in a nonsurgical procedure, and quite another to find a qualified, reputable physician to entrust your face to. As anyone who's enjoyed an extraordinary dinner one night and suffered through a miserable one the next will tell you, technique is everything. It's exactly the same with a cosmetic procedure. The ingredients might not be different, but it's the skill of the technician that will leave you with mediocre or amazing results.

Considering that I administer more Botox and collagen injections than any other physician in this country (this isn't merely a boast, but a fact that the makers of both treatments have publicly stated), I think I'm something of an authority on what makes a physician a good choice for Botox, collagen, Restylane, silicone, and any other type of procedure that can quickly and easily give your skin a beautiful boost. Here, now, are my top ten questions to ask your potential physician.

1. What is the physician trained in? Is he or she trained in dermatology (which is the ideal) or something completely unrelated, like hematology?

2. Is the physician board-certified in that specialty? You'd be surprised at how many physicians are not board-certified, so that you miss out on the extra training and knowledge this certification represents.

3. What specific training has the physician had in the types of procedures he or she administers? Additional training isn't mandatory, but it's always a bonus.

4. Are cosmetic dermatology treatments the primary focus of the physician's practice? Or is a procedure

like Botox something that he or she does only occasionally?

5. What kind of results can I expect? An honest physician will tell you what results are realistic.

6. How many treatments will I need to achieve my desired results?

7. How often will I have to come in for maintenance?

8. What are the potential side effects from my chosen procedure?

9. Does the physician have any "before" and "after" pictures that he or she can share with you? It's always helpful to see real people who have undergone such procedures, even in Polaroid photos.

10. What is this going to cost me? Ask for a detailed list of prices, including all those hidden fees. Keep in mind that a "name" physician who practices in a large city might be pricier than one from a smaller town.

No doubt about it, we are a country that cares about good looks just as much as we do about moral fiber. We are also a country that is aging—the estimated 76 million baby boomers born between 1946 and 1964 are steadily marching into middle age, and unlike generations before, these men and women refuse to let the passage of time change how they feel about themselves. And with the vast array of rejuvenating cosmetic treatments at their disposal, they certainly don't have to.

four

: Bring on the Botox :

'm often asked what I consider to be the greatest advance in cosmetic dermatology. Without hesitation I say, "Botox." The advent of treating wrinkles with Botox injections has allowed doctors like myself to treat conditions that in the past not even plastic surgery could remedy. Don't like the way your forehead stays furrowed long after you've stopped worrying? Then shoot those lines into oblivion. What about those little lines around your eyes that are still in existence despite your fanatical use of eye cream? Shoot some Botox there, too. And whatever happened to your regal neck? Yes, Botox will bring back your beloved neck as well. All this improvement with no recovery period, minimal pain, and extremely natural results.

Botox has many uses, but its claim to fame is how well it smooths dynamic wrinkles, also known as "wrinkles in motion." These lines are most often found across the forehead, between the brows, and around the eyes. Constant frowning is one sure way to get them, but any sort of movement will bring them on, including laughing heartily and squinting at your computer screen. In other words, just being alive brings them on. What happens over time is that the line morphs from a "wrinkle in motion" to the more dreaded "wrinkle at rest." Like it or not, that little guy is there to stay.

For a substance with such dramatic properties for beautification, Botox has a much publicized controversial background. Botox, or "botulinum toxin type A," is a highly purified derivative of the toxin that in much, much larger doses could be hazardous. When used for cosmetic purposes—or wrinkle zapping—the purified toxin is diluted and injected into the facial muscles. Almost instantly, the toxin blocks the nerve impulses that control muscle movement by restricting the patient's ability to contract the facial muscles. No contraction of the muscle equals no movement of the skin lying over it, and no movement equals no wrinkles. A smoothing effect is seen while the patient is still in the exam chair, and improvement continues over the following couple of days. The result lasts approximately three to six months, at which point most patients gradually return to their original state of wrinkling.

Of the seven existing forms of the botulinum toxin, type A is most studied and most used, and is the only one approved by the FDA for the cosmetic treatment of frown lines. Myobloc, manufactured by Elan Pharmaceuticals, is another paralyzing agent, derived from botulinum type B. It is used very similarly to Botox, but its FDA-approved only for cervical dystonia, involuntary contractions of the neck and shoulders. However, the potential of Myobloc as a cosmetic treatment is starting to emerge, and more information should come within the next couple of years.

The American Society for Aesthetic Plastic Surgery (ASAPS) recently released statistics on all the surgical and nonsurgical cosmetic procedures performed last year. In the case of Botox, the figures were mind-boggling. It was ranked as the most often requested nonsurgical cosmetic procedure, with more than 1.6 million Americans treated in just one year. Of that figure, more than 86 percent of the patients were female, and the remaining 13 percent were male. (The other four top nonsurgical cosmetic procedures were chemical peels, collagen injections, microdermabrasion, and laser hair removal.)

The immobilizing property that makes Botox sound potentially morbid is also what makes it an incredible drug. During the 1980s, researchers discovered that it was of tremendous benefit to patients suffering from involuntary muscle spasms associated with illnesses such as cerebral palsy. Compared with the other treatments available at the time, such as muscle relaxants, Botox was found to be the most effective, since it worked quickly and had minimal side effects. In 1989 the FDA approved Botox for the treatment of strabismus (commonly known as "crossed eyes") and blepharospasm (involuntary winking). The following year Botox was granted another approval, this time for cervical dystonia.

The story of how Botox was transformed from a medical drug to one with myriad cosmetic benefits is as fascinating as Botox itself. An ophthalmologist in Canada, Dr. Jean Carruthers, noticed that patients she was treating with Botox were not only seeing an improvement in their medical conditions but also finding that the wrinkles in the surrounding areas were virtually disappearing. Intrigued by this development, Dr. Carruthers mentioned it to her husband, who happened to be a dermatologist. Just as intrigued, he began to try out Botox on his patients—starting with his thirty-year-old receptionist, who had deep creases between her eyebrows— and he arrived at the same conclusion as his wife. A few years later, in 1990, the first medical paper was written on the potential of Botox as a significant aid in the field of cosmetic dermatology, bringing Botox greater recognition and acceptance among cosmetic dermatologists.

The buzz on Botox started to spread, and I became among the first in my field to participate in this exciting development. At the time, a lot of my patients were frightened of Botox and its perceived dangers. And to be honest, I can understand these fears. There's something slightly alarming about telling patients that I'm going to erase their wrinkles with a shot of something that originates as a toxin!

The fact is that nobody has been harmed by Botox or even had an allergic reaction to it—much less died from it. Research has found that in humans, a lethal injection would consist of 2,500 to 3,000 units of Botox. For patients suffering from the muscle spasms associated with cerebral palsy, to mention just one example, dosages as high as 1,000 units are used quite routinely. And when Botox is used for cosmetic reasons the average dosage is—drumroll, please—up to 75 units. That's paltry and insignificant and, most important to you, *extremely* safe.

Once their concerns were assuaged, the next question was the all-important "How will I look?" Would patients look strange and oddly frozen? Would others detect their little secret? Even today, one of the biggest misconceptions about Botox is that it will eliminate all facial expression. This theory is so widespread that even Hollywood directors have put their two cents into the Botox debate, arguing that Botox has robbed their actresses of the ability to emote. I've certainly seen my fair share of expressionless faces, but with as much Botox as I administer in a day, I can vouch for how natural Botox can look. Proper technique, an artistic eye, and a conservative approach should result in the patients who look like themselves, only refreshed and rejuvenated.

Almost a decade after Botox arrived on the scene, a spotless record of success has finally earned it the FDA's approval for treating moderate to severe wrinkling in the glabellar lines, commonly referred to as frown lines. These two grooves are parallel to each other above the bridge of the nose; with time, they tend to become deeper and more prominent. Of course, the potential of Botox isn't limited to this one area. The FDA requires that a drug prove its safety and effectiveness through clinical trials; and for Botox, which has many uses, proof must be presented, and approval is awarded, for each application. For example, Botox is extremely effective at erasing (albeit temporarily) crow's feet and the bands on the forehead, so those are the areas that will probably receive the next approval for cosmetic use. Approval for treating back spasms and migraine headaches might be next. In the meantime, physicians can use Botox however they see fit. This is called off-label usage, and it's a practice that is perfectly legal as long as the FDA has approved the drug for something.

For now, this validation is a huge step toward bringing greater acceptance and understanding of the many conditions that can be treated with Botox. I was one of the handful of physicians who conducted the clinical trials that led to the FDA's decision, and I believe that this cosmetic equivalent of the Good Housekeeping Seal of Approval will allow patients to feel more comfortable seeking treatment with Botox. The FDA's approval has also permitted Allergan, Inc., the manufacturer of Botox, to finally promote it as a valid treatment for frown lines. (And there's no escaping the $50 million magazine and television ad campaign touting the cosmetic prowess of Botox. Allergan, it seems, wants to spread the word on Botox.)

With this newfound respect, however, comes a dangerous misconception that since Botox is a relatively quick and simple procedure, it can be done anywhere, by anyone. This couldn't be farther from the truth. The fact that Botox injections can be administered in less than thirty minutes doesn't make the procedure less serious than, say, LASIK eye correction. The physicians who are best suited to administer Botox are trained, board-certified cosmetic dermatologists and plastic surgeons who have extensive experience with Botox and an advanced understanding of facial anatomy. Surely you've heard of Botox parties, where a group of people mingle in a salon or similar setting, alcohol is served, and Botox is administered in another room by a physician. If a complication were to arise, would you want a bunch of your tipsy friends cheering you on? Probably not.

Now for that crucial question: How does it look? If there's one word that sums up the result attained with Botox, it's "normal." "Rested" and "rejuvenated" are other good adjectives, as are "refreshed" and "replenished." Quite simply, you look much the same, but better. The areas that needed smoothing are smoothed; the parts that were sagging are now uplifted. If you don't personally know someone who's been injected with Botox (although that is a little hard to believe), I would suggest that you turn on your television. Or go to the movies. Or pick up a fashion magazine. I can't say with total certainty just how many celebrities have jumped on the Botox bandwagon, but trust me when I say that if you're over forty and in the public eye, you've probably gone in for a little injection rejuvenation.

: The Botox Face-Lift :

One of the most exciting uses of Botox is one I pioneered in 1997, when I discovered that by injecting Botox into the cords of a patient's neck, I could get results that resembled those from a face-lift. Allow me to explain. A face-lift, despite its name, treats conditions that are exclusive to the lower half of the face, such as loose skin on the cheeks, a softened jawline, thickened neck bands, and a crinkled neck. Those who have a significant amount of sagging fat in the face and neck would get great results from a face-lift, not for people who aren't yet at such an advanced stage of aging. For them, Botox in the neck would be the procedure of choice.

This use of Botox is so instantly and dramatically effective that you truly have to see it to believe it. A few quick injections of Botox in the cords of the neck, and presto, the bands in the neck become less prominent, the lines there disappear, the jowls are diminished, and even the outer corners of the mouth get picked up slightly. Another plus: there's practically no pain associated with injecting the neck. It's a wonderfully satisfying way to use Botox, and patients, even those who are initially skeptical about treating the neck, are thrilled with the results. I must stress, however, that because the muscles on the lower half of the face are not as clearly defined as those on the upper part of the face, it might be difficult for an inexperienced practitioner to deliver good results in this area.

Nothing will stop aging permanently, not even plastic surgery, so it's not uncommon for me to see patients who've already had a face-lift (or two) and would like to get a slight lift without having to undergo surgery again. When they hear that Botox will save them another trip to the plastic surgeon's office, they're very relieved. They're also being smart. Constantly pulling the face back will not make you look any younger and will only give you that dreaded wind-tunnel effect. (You know the look. It's the one that keeps people whispering after the person has left the room.)

: The Botox Brow-Lift :

The eyes are said to be the windows to the soul, and while this is a cliché, it might explain why nearly every patient is concerned with the appearance of his or her eyes. Even patients in their twenties will ask me if a plastic surgery procedure, such as an eye-lift, is the answer to their particular problems. Before

I answer this, I first hand them a mirror and ask them to point out what it is about their eyes that is bothering them. If the problem is excess skin above the eyelid or bags below the eyes, then surgery can definitely help, but so can Botox.

When the muscles over the brows are injected with Botox, that area immediately lifts, bringing with it any excess skin that is hanging over the eyes. Suddenly, the eyes seem bigger, more open, and brighter, almost as if a light had just been turned on overhead. I refer to this phenomenon as a nonsurgical brow lift. After the patients are handed the mirror again to observe the results on one side of the face, they happily exclaim that they had no idea they could have such a result without surgery. It's not too far-fetched to predict that Botox could someday replace surgical brow-lifts—it's hard to dispute such dramatic benefits, reaped with so little pain and zero downtime.

Those new to Botox are fascinated by how a needle can reshape the brows, in the process opening up the eyes and subtracting years from their age. Keep in mind, though, that as thrilling as the brow-lift can be, the brows are a tricky area to treat correctly. There's a fine line between rejuvenating the face and freezing it into submission, and only an experienced doctor can avoid an undesirable result. Trust only a physician who is reputed to know the difference.

My approach to each patient is customized. I start by assessing not just the patient's forehead lines but also his or her overall facial structure. Those elements give me enough information to map out a plan. Let's say that a patient's forehead lines are very pronounced but her brow is naturally low. In that instance I wouldn't attempt to completely erase every single line, since in the process I risk lowering the brow even further, leaving the patient with an eye area that looks closed (or simply with less space to apply eye shadow). It's a delicate balance, since totally paralyzing (and in the process, softening) the forehead muscles takes away the ability to elevate the brows. I feel it's more important to have open eyes and a few lines on the forehead than a totally smooth but lowered brow.

: The Eyes Have It :

There's nothing like Botox for treating crow's feet, those little lines that hover at the outer corner of each eye. These lines are known as dynamic wrinkles, or wrinkles in motion, and their existence is related to the constant movement of that part of the face. As I said earlier, Botox is, without question, the treatment of choice for any type of movement-induced wrinkling. Plastic surgery does nothing for crow's feet but pull them tighter. Collagen injections will make them appear softer when the patient isn't animated, but daily facial expressions will bring them back in no time. As for treating them with lasers, you will see an improvement, but it comes at the price of two weeks of recovery time and a risk of permanent changes in your pigmentation.

A fatty deposit under the eyes is best treated with surgery, but I've found that a lot of patients, particularly those who are under forty years old, mistake a bulge right under the eye for fat. This bulge is actually an overworked muscle, and, believe it or not, a touch of Botox injected there will soften it. As bizarre as injecting your eye with Botox sounds, it is very safe to do so. The only consequence is that this can round out the eye shape. (A lot of my Asian patients actually consider this a perk.) Bottom line: if you love your almond-shaped eyes, then I wouldn't recommend this for you.

: Botox All Around :

One of the reasons why I'm such a believer in Botox is that its immense versatility is unmatched. New uses for it seem to surface daily, and it's so satisfying when patients see results from Botox that they never dreamed of obtaining in such a short visit. Following are a few examples of Botox's scope.

: Migraines :

It's been proved that Botox helps with migraine headaches, a debilitating condition. The reason isn't exactly clear, but I suspect that the muscle-relaxing effect of Botox has something to do with it. Another theory is that Botox has a positive effect on the pain transmitters in the face. A few years ago I treated a patient who I thought was exaggerating when she said her headache had disappeared immediately after she was injected with Botox. Today, however, I'm a believer in this application. Recently another patient told me that her crippling headaches had kept her home from work for two weeks and that to her, Botox was truly heaven-sent. Even one of the nurses in my Miami office uses Botox for this purpose; her headaches are so severe that she often has to turn off the lights in her office and rest her head. For many, the instant relief that Botox delivers in just a shot or two—with relief lasting as long as four months—is far more desirable than taking an endless stream of pain medication. Of course, no one complains about the side benefits!

: Excessive Sweating :

It doesn't classify as a cosmetic problem in the traditional sense, but profuse sweating (hyperhidrosis) is a big issue for a lot of people. Picture a supermodel walking down a runway with an armpit stain or a businessman sealing a deal with a clammy handshake and it becomes clear why many people are desperate for a solution. As it happens, the neurotransmitter (acetylcholine) that Botox affects in the face is the same one that triggers the sweat glands under the arms and in the palms of the hands, the soles of the feet, and the forehead. Treating these areas with Botox temporarily reduces or even halts sweat production, with results lasting anywhere from six to eight months.

: Chest :

Isn't it odd to see a perfectly unlined face above a chest full of lines? I think so, and so do the patients whom I've treated in that area. I remember one patient in particular gushing about the thrill of waking up in the morning and not having a network of lines running in all directions.

: Odds and Ends :

We already know that aging causes everything to droop, but the nose, too? Unfortunately, this is also true, and as a result the nose tends to appear longer. A tiny amount of Botox injected in the tip of the nose can help relax the muscle that is causing the droop. Another consequence of aging is loss of fat and muscle, and in the chin this manifests as a dimpled "cobblestone" effect. Again, a shot or two of Botox restores it quite well.

: Side Effects :

By now you're probably thinking that Botox has to have a downside. As with any other procedure, whether cosmetic or not, side effects are always a concern. In the case of Botox, the most common side effects are headaches, drooping of the eyebrow (brow ptosis), drooping of the eyelid (eyelid ptosis), double vision, and paralysis of the wrong muscles. Expect most of these side effects to clear up on their own within a few weeks. The only exception is brow ptosis, which can last as long as the Botox. Bruising at the site of the injection is another possible side effect. However, choosing an experienced physician lessens your chances of winding up with any of these side effects.

: Tips of the Botox Trade :

1. Certain vitamins and medications, such as vitamin E and aspirin, can make you more prone to bruising at the injection site. Avoid them for approximately 10 days before being treated with Botox.
2. It's important to remain upright for a minimum of two hours following treatment to ensure that Botox doesn't migrate. One of my new patients came prepared with an antisnooze gadget created for drivers that gets tucked behind the ear. It works by emitting a loud buzzing sound whenever it senses that the head is lowering. The best part of this story is that her mother, also a patient, had given it to her!
3. Excessive smiling and frowning are what brought you to seek Botox in the first place. Oddly enough, though, you'll have to do a lot of both immediately after the treatment to ensure that the Botox binds properly.

: The Botox Consultation :

I've found that while patients are all too aware of their problem areas, they're usually at a loss as to which procedure will help restore their looks. This confusion is quite understandable, and it's one of the reasons why the consultation is an invaluable factor in ultimately having a fulfilling experience. When I meet patients for the first time, I'm not only listening to what they're saying but also observing their facial expressions. That in itself will tell me a lot. If, for example, a patient is constantly pursing his or her lips when speaking, then I know that the lines on the upper and lower lips are due to muscular contractions, making this patient an ideal candidate for Botox. I would then explain how tiny drops of Botox would simply relax this area, not paralyze it. Afterward, I might suggest a follow-up with a peel or a laser treatment. The combination of treatments will ensure that the area remains smooth for even longer.

: What a Pain :

Patients often ask me if Botox is a painful procedure. As with any type of pain, different people feel it differently. Also, I've found that people are sometimes mainly afraid of the unknown, and once they have the treatment they're surprised at how tolerable it was. Some other people have a chronic fear of needles. I show them how tiny the needles are, rather like acupuncture needles, and this comforts them. But trust me when I say that Botox is the best wash-and-wear procedure out there. It can even be done on the night of a party! I recommend that a patient use a topical anesthetic cream, usually EMLA, for thirty minutes before the procedure. This extra step is worthwhile because it definitely decreases pain during the procedure.

The procedure itself, consisting of a few pricks throughout the face, lasts no longer than fifteen minutes. I remember a new patient who was greatly afraid of the pain and would talk of nothing else. I asked her to sit back and relax, and minutes later she was giddy over how comfortable the procedure had been. She even exclaimed that having her eyebrows tweezed was far more painful. After the very last shot is injected, we place ice packs over the face to decrease any discomfort and to help prevent any bruising that might come later.

: The Fear Factor :

Patients often ask me if Botox will cause their muscles to atrophy. Studies have shown that approximately six to eight months after stopping Botox, 80 percent of the muscle mass goes back to normal. Bottom line: you're not going to lose control over your muscles. Some patients are even concerned about how Botox will affect their respiration, but I can guarantee that the amount of Botox used cosmetically will in no way affect this.

: Is There Such a Thing as Too Much Botox? :

The only way that too much Botox becomes a problem is when an excessive amount is injected in one sitting, resulting in a frozen forehead, lowered brow, and possible drooping of the eyelid. Over time, a very small group of patients will develop immunity to Botox, meaning that subsequent treatments won't have an effect.

What can Botox treat?

1. furrowed eyebrows
2. forehead lines

3. lifts brows, for a nonsurgical "brow-lift"
4. crow's feet
5. under-eye bulge, to open the eyes
6. lines and bands in neck
7. vertical "smoker's" lines that run above and below the lips
8. vertical "marionette" lines that run from the outside corner of the mouth to the chin
9. dimpling on chin
10. prominent jowling
11. lines on chest
12. excessive sweating
13. painful headaches

What can't Botox do?

1. enlarge lips
2. smooth nasolabial folds
3. add volume to cheeks

Whether you'd never heard of Botox or have been contemplating it for a while, remember that Botox delivers maximum results with the least recuperation possible. You'll still look like yourself, only a more refreshed, more energized version.

five

: Filler Up :

The world of cosmetic dermatology is littered with awkward moments—who doesn't remember groaning at Goldie Hawn's overinflated lips in the movie *The First Wives' Club*? With such an exaggerated image, it's easy to see why the concept of correcting facial flaws by injecting them with a foreign substance can seem like modern-day nuttiness. In reality, however, the category of "fillers" is an extremely valid one, as fillers are the most effective way to improve a long list of skin woes, from softening the appearance of wrinkles and scars to restoring youthful volume to the face and even giving lips that sexy oomph you've only dreamed about. Fillers should be in everyone's antiaging arsenal.

The concept of filler materials dates back to the nineteenth century, when researchers discovered that fat taken from a patient's body was ideal for fixing facial defects. By the early 1900s, paraffin—yes, as in wax—was being experimented with, although it fell out of favor twenty years later. The 1940s saw a fascination with silicone fillers, but that fad came to an end when it was discovered that silicone had an unfortunate tendency to migrate from the intended location when injected incorrectly. (Improved versions of silicone are in use today, and I'll discuss them later in this chapter.)

In the early 1970s, a team of researchers at Stanford University in California began tinkering with bovine (cow-based) collagen. The results were very promising, and finally, in 1977, the first bovine collagen injection—with the trade name Zyderm—hit the market. The FDA granted approval in 1981, and today Zyderm maintains its unrivaled popularity. Two other versions of bovine collagen, Zyderm II and Zyplast, soon followed. Depending on the patient's needs, any of the three can be used, either exclusively or in combination.

By now you're probably asking yourself, "Why from cows?" First, the collagen found in cows is very similar to human collagen and as a result, only an estimated 3 percent of the population is allergic to it. A series of tests spaced over a four-week period usually rule out the possibility of an allergic reaction; in these tests, it's been found that only one in 1,000 patients will experience the redness and swelling at the site of the injection associated with an allergic reaction. Fortunately, the reaction always clears up on its own and doesn't affect your general health. Second, and perhaps more important, bovine collagen delivers an extremely natural result that so far has proved difficult to replicate with a synthetic substance or even a human one.

As remarkable as bovine collagen is, however, it does have disadvantages. The possibility of an allergic reaction, however small, still means that some people are not able to use it. Also, once it is injected the body quickly breaks it down, and in three to six months most of the effect will have disappeared.

It's easy to see how collagen injections can soon add up to an expensive quick fix!

Not surprisingly, attempts have been made to discover the "perfect" filler. This endeavor has proved to be as challenging as finding the fountain of youth. Such a filler would have to satisfy a list of requirements to be classified as perfect. It should be long-lasting, look natural, be derived from a material that doesn't pose the risk of an allergic reaction, and be easy to administer. Currently, there are a lot of promising options that meet some of these requirements, but not all. We will be examining these options in this chapter, as well as presenting what you can expect to see in the very near future.

The American Society for Aesthetic Plastic Surgery reports that more than a million collagen injections were administered in the United States in 2001, an increase of 85 percent from 2000. To truly gauge how popular collagen injections now are, consider that the figures for 2001 reflect a 216 percent increase in injections administered since 1997. Obviously, collagen injections are working out wonderfully for a lot of people.

: Are Fillers for You? :

A good way to determine whether you would benefit from a filler material is to study your reflection in the mirror and ask yourself the following questions: Do you have deep lines from the corner of the nose to the mouth? (These folds are also called smile lines, except that they're nothing to smile about, are they?) What about your forehead? Do you see a series of horizontal lines? Now concentrate on your mouth for a moment—do you have a multitude of tiny vertical lines above and below your lips, or are the corners of your mouth turned down slightly, as if you were sulking? While you're looking at your lips, consider whether you would like to replace some of the volume that time has taken away. Finally, does your face seem hollow and devoid of the roundness of your youth?

If, when you step away from the mirror, you have answered yes to at least one of those questions, then you're most likely an ideal candidate for treatment with a filler material.

: Lip Service :

Many people are concerned about the appearance of their mouth, and understandably so. This is an area where aging rears its ugly head: the lips shrink with age and the borders of the mouth, which function very much like a frame, tend to lose definition. The corners of the mouth, meanwhile, turn downward, giving the face a sad appearance and further contributing to the marionette lines (oral commissures) that run down to the chin.

My preferred method for restoring the integrity of the mouth is to inject a filler material like collagen right along the borders of the lips. A lot of women are afraid that this technique will give them lips that are too plumped—no doubt thinking of *The First Wives' Club*—but I assure them that if the procedure is done properly, using only small amounts of a filler material, this will not be the case. A great side benefit of this technique is that the corners of the lips are lifted, bringing back that youthful smile. I'd even say that you could easily bring the lips back to their appearance of twenty years ago!

Another common complaint has to do with the annoying "lipstick bleed" lines (formally known as perioral lines) that hover directly above and below the lips. I always tell my patients that although I could fill in these tiny lines with a filler—and this approach would solve the problem for a lot of patients—the perfectionist in me feels that this is akin to painting only a portion of a room. To truly improve this area I would suggest we fill in the borders of the lips as well. This technique will act as a foundation for the filler that is already injected in the upper and lower lip lines, helping it not to be broken down as quickly.

Almost daily, patients enter my office clutching a photo of the lips of their dreams. (I probably have enough of these photos in my office to fill another whole book!) More often than not, these fantasy lips are full and luscious—Angelina Jolie is the poster child for this phenomenon. Again, I try to convey to the patient that while the lips can be enhanced, the end result still has to be appropriate for her own face. Nothing is worse than seeing the lips coming through the door ten seconds before the person does.

First, I suggest that we subtly inject filler to outline the lips. Quite often this step gives enough of a change and the patient can choose to stop there. But if patients decide that they do indeed want something fuller, I achieve it by filling in the entire lip with the chosen filler. My goal is to have the patient leave my office with lips that look as if she had been born with them. An interesting footnote is the question of which lip should be fuller: top or bottom? The upper lip is often in greater need of plumping, since it tends to lose the most volume, but I like the bottom lip to be slightly larger so that it forms a nice platform on which the top lip can rest.

: Eye on the Prize :

Dark circles under the eyes contribute greatly to a drained, fatigued look, and nearly everyone wants to know what can be done about them. The purplish hue is due to dilated blood vessels that lie just below the surface and show through the area's thin, translucent skin. Elevating the under-eye area with a filler can create a new, thicker layer of skin that can help to camouflage these blood vessels. This procedure will also fill in the groove around the eyes, making it a whole lot smoother.

: Scar Face :

Accidents and disease can leave behind unpleasant souvenirs in the form of scarring. Luckily, certain types of scars can be filled in with a filler material. A quick way to see if a specific scar would benefit from a filler is to hold the skin between the fingers and pull it taut. If the skin smooths out with this action, then it's probably a good candidate for filling. Other types of scars, like "ice pick" scars, cannot be successfully treated with filler materials.

: What Can't a Filler Do? :

By definition, a filler does not tighten the skin, so saggy jowls cannot be treated. Fillers are somewhat helpful in filling in dynamic wrinkles, such as those commonly found on the forehead and around the eyes, but Botox is much better suited for this, since the constant flexing of the muscle will quickly bring back the wrinkle.

I wish I could say that fillers can make those dreaded large pores a condition of the past. No such luck, as the structure of pores would result in the filler material's being pushed right out.

: How Many Filler Materials Are Available Today? :

The list of filler materials available today is long and ever-changing, but bovine collagen injections are still considered the gold standard among fillers. In addition to having the longest track record of safety, bovine collagen is available in two forms, assuring that virtually every area in need of augmentation can be treated. However, researchers are working like mad to knock bovine collagen off its very high horse, and innovations in this category might just accomplish that feat.

Here is a complete overview of fillers on the market today in the United States, as well as those soon to arrive.

: Biological Fillers :

Biological fillers are materials derived from humans or animals that are naturally degraded by the body.

Bovine Collagen

Anyone who is considering collagen injections for the first time wants to know the following: Is the procedure painful? Will the collagen be bumpy under the skin? How long will the results last? And most important, will I look so bad afterward that I'll have to miss that great party?

For starters, collagen injections are one of the most comfortable procedures out there, thanks to the lidocaine, a local anesthetic, that's already premixed in the syringe. To make the entire process completely painless, a patient can choose to numb the area that will be treated with a thick coating of a cream that also contains lidocaine. Some patients choose to undergo the procedure without this extra step, while others happily ask for it and use the additional thirty minutes of waiting time to catch up on their magazines. The cream is then removed, the procedure is performed, and the skin remains numb for approximately an hour afterward.

Some patients say they see results immediately; for others, it might take three to four days for the collagen to settle into the skin. It's quite common for patients to have some redness on the first day, but that is easily camouflaged with makeup. On average, patients need to return every four months to maintain the effects. This doesn't mean that the collagen has completely disappeared, but in order to maintain the original results, a touch-up is necessary. The good news is that those who start collagen treatments while still fairly young—for instance, in their thirties—may obtain nearly permanent results due to the constant stimulation of their own collagen.

Aside from everything you already know about bovine collagen, it's important to note that you suffer no risk of contracting the "mad cow disease" that has plagued certain European countries. The company that manufactures Zyderm and Zyplast, the McGhan Medical Corporation, uses cows that have been raised on an isolated ranch in California. So erase that concern from your list!

- *Zyderm I and Zyderm II:* A non-cross-linked bovine collagen that is ideal for treating superficial wrinkles like horizontal forehead lines, crow's feet, and shallow scars. As I mentioned earlier, these injections are premixed with lidocaine, a pain reliever, so that the procedure is minimally painful. Zyderm II is a more concentrated version of bovine collagen. Your physician can help you determine which version is right for you.
- *Zyplast:* This is cross-linked bovine collagen, meaning that the substance is thicker and more durable than Zyderm. It is ideal for deeper wrinkles and furrows, nasolabial folds, and deep scars, and for enhancing the lip line.

Human Collagen: Cosmoderm and Cosmoplast

These two materials, also from McGhan Medical, are perfect examples of innovations in filler materials. Made of collagen that is derived from infant foreskin cells, Cosmoderm and Cosmoplast are considered the ideal form of human collagen. This form is ideal because it poses no risk of an allergic reaction and therefore eliminates the need for skin testing before treatment—a great bonus for people who are too impatient to wait four weeks for test results before being treated. Also, its source ensures an incomparable purity.

It's difficult to state with any degree of accuracy just how long the results with this filler last. Cosmetic treatments that involve human collagen have not been widely used, and therefore few statistics are available. However, considering that the human collagen in Cosmoderm and Cosmoplast has the same composition as bovine collagen, it might be safe to say that the duration should be similar to that of Zyderm and Zyplast. And, as with bovine collagen injections, the syringe comes premixed with lidocaine for minimal discomfort. Applications of Cosmoderm I and II are similar to those of Zyderm I and II. Cosmoplast is equivalent to Zyplast and can be used similarly.

As of the writing of this book, this material is not yet available anywhere. Most likely it will be available in late 2002 or early in 2003.

Human Injectable Tissue

CYMETRA

A mixture of collagen, elastin, and glycosaminoglycans—three substances that are found naturally in the dermis of the skin—Cymetra is derived from donated human cadaver skin. An advantage of Cymetra is that it poses no risk of an allergic reaction, and therefore the need for skin testing is eliminated. A disadvantage is that the injection is more painful than bovine collagen, as there is no anesthetic in the syringe. Also, because Cymetra is available in just one thickness, it lacks the versatility of other fillers. In general, its use is limited to the treatment of superficial lines and wrinkles.

Isolagen is a material with various benefits, but speediness is definitely not among them. First, fibroblasts, the skin cells that produce collagen, are retrieved from behind the patient's ear and sent to an outside lab, where they are allowed to multiply. After the cells are returned to the physician, the patient has just a short window of opportunity for the cells to be injected into the skin. If too much time elapses, the cells will die off and be rendered useless. It's important to remember that since fibroblasts, not collagen, are injected into the skin, the patient does not leave the office with visible results. Actually, it could take as long as four months after the treatment for enough collagen to be synthesized so that a change is seen in a patient's wrinkles.

If you're still interested in pursuing treatments with Isolagen, there's a catch: it's not going to be available for at least three years. Isolagen was available from 1996 to 1999 but had to be taken off the market because of an FDA classification issue that had nothing to do with safety.

Hyaluronic Acids

Almost daily, the question "What's new?" comes up in conversations with my patients, and frequently this inquiry is directed toward the latest filler materials. Innovation is always intriguing to patients, but they are equally interested in learning about new fillers that are long-lasting and safe. My reply is that, of all the new injectable fillers that are on the horizon, the hyaluronic acid family of products is the most exciting.

Hyaluronic acid is a polysaccharide, or natural sugar, that is crucial to the healthy functioning of the human body. The skin houses the vast majority of hyaluronic acid, with the remainder found in the muscles and skeleton. Its primary function is to provide volume and pliability to the skin and it plays a crucial role in cell growth. Interestingly enough, hyaluronic acid is commonly used in moisturizers and other cosmetics, as it is wonderfully efficient at holding on to water. An often-mentioned characteristic of hyaluronic acid is its capacity to bind water up to a thousand times its volume. This property makes it ideal as a filler material, for even while a hyaluronic acid filler is being naturally degraded, what remains of the filler attracts water from the body, and that function allows it to hold its shape even longer.

In the 1960s, the first hyaluronic acid product was used for eye surgery. Today there are two families of such fillers currently available for cosmetic use. The first is created in a lab while the other is derived from an animal source.

Nonanimal Hyaluronic Acid

In 1996, the biotechnology company Q-Med of Sweden created a genetically engineered version of hyaluronic acid in the form of a clear gel called NASHA (nonanimal stabilized hyaluronic acid). This technology, which was found to be compatible with human skin, was used to make Restylane, an injectable filler that can be injected like collagen. Restylane has been used extensively in Europe, Canada, and South America for years, and the results so far have been extremely positive.

Several years after the introduction of Restylane, the company came up with two other versions: Restylane Fine Lines and Perlane. Both have the same chemical composition as the original product, but the thickness varies among the three. Restylane Fine Lines can be used for superficial lines anywhere on the face, such as those lines above and below the lip that lipstick always seems to bleed into. The thickest of the three materials is Perlane, which can be used to sculpt the face, that is, enhance the cheekbones and soften a sharp chin. (A result of aging, this pointiness reminds me of a witch's chin. Not very attractive, right?) Men, too, are great candidates for Perlane and seek it for creating a stronger jawline. It's even been used successfully to replace the tissue on the temples that diminishes with age. Of course, deeper lines such as nasolabial folds and scars in the cheeks are also candidates for treatment with the Restylane group of products, as are the lips. With all three fillers, I can tailor my injections to target the specific problems of the skin.

I predict that the Restylane family of fillers will revolutionize the area of cosmetic dermatology and ultimately give collagen injections a real run for their money. I say this for two reasons. First, these materials are extremely versatile—I can fill in lines as I do with collagen, as well as restore volume to the face as I used to do with fat, minus the surgical procedure. Oddly enough, many people are too thin these days and don't have any extra fat to spare! Second, one of my favorite characteristics of Restylane is that a small amount of it can go very far. In other words, one syringe of Restylane allows me to treat a greater area than one syringe of collagen. For the patient, this means that a treatment with Restylane can be less expensive than collagen.

Allergic reactions to Restylane aren't a significant concern, but since it is genetically engineered in a lab, small amounts of protein might remain in the mixture. This has been found to cause an allergic reaction in one out of more than 6,000 people. I believe that as the manufacturing process is refined, this figure will get even lower.

As one of the few dermatologists chosen to conduct the FDA clinical trials for Restylane in the United States, I've had ample opportunity to work with this filler. The first results are already showing that Restylane lasts almost 60 percent longer than collagen. On average, a patient can expect an improvement from six months to as long as a year. I've also found that

Restylane delivers smoother results than collagen, with significantly less bruising and bumpiness. And, of course, the fact that no skin testing is required is very appealing to many patients. The only downside that I can think of is that it's a slightly more painful injection, but a topical anesthetic cream should help ease any discomfort.

Now for the bad news: the Restylane group of products is not available in the United States—yet. At present, the FDA trials for Restylane are being completed, and approval is expected in early 2003.

ANIMAL-DERIVED HYALURONIC ACID

Hyaluronic acid is also abundant in animals, and researchers have turned to roosters—yes, roosters, since their combs are a rich source of hyaluronic acid—to come up with another source. Hylaform, also known as Hylan Gel or Hylan B, is such a filler. Since hyaluronic acid has the same chemical composition in all animals, this rooster-derived version poses no hazard of triggering an allergic reaction, and hence no skin testing is required.

Like Restylane, this source of hyaluronic acid is also available in three forms: Hylaform and Hylaform Plus, both of which function like Perlane, as well as Hylaform Fine Lines. As of the writing of this book, the FDA has not started working on the necessary trials to grant approval for use in the United States. Most likely, Restylane will be available first, and in my opinion it will be a more popular product. Its use in Europe has shown that Restylane lasts longer than Hylaform, and the fact that it is derived from a nonanimal source is a definite advantage.

Fat

There are more ways to inject fat than there are recipes for making stew. Although this filler has been popular for more than a hundred years, positive results remain highly dependent on the experience of the physician as well as on the technique used. First, fat is removed from the patient, usually from the lower body. Some is injected into the face on the same day. The remainder is kept frozen until the patient returns to the office for another treatment. Some physicians like to treat their patients once a month over a period of several months with small doses of fat. Others, meanwhile, opt to inject megadoses of fat in just one session. The downside to the latter option is the swelling and longer recuperation time; the upside is that the results appear to be long-lasting. Smaller dosages do deliver good results, but this technique doesn't seem to deliver the long-lasting results that larger doses do. The bottom line is that every physician has his or her own method of injecting fat, and accordingly, the results will vary.

Fat injections are great for enhancing volume and giving the face contours, but they're not as effective for fine lines. Also, there is usually some swelling and bruising, as the needle is larger than the one used for hyaluronic acid or collagen injections. Traditionally the fat is injected right into the patient's facial fat. Some doctors are experimenting with injecting fat into the muscle, but so far I have not seen enough positive results to be convinced of the viability of this technique. Overall, I think that the results with fat can be semipermanent in some people and will last even less than collagen in other people. Finally, certain areas, like smile lines, seem to show greater improvement than areas like the lips.

Human Fascia

"Fascia" is a medical term used to describe the thick sheets of connective tissue that line muscles. Fascia has been used safely as a surgical implant for years. Recently, Fascian, an injectable particulate form of fascia derived from human cadavers, has become available. With Fascian, freeze-dried particles of this connective tissue are combined with a local anesthetic to create a dense suspension, and that is then implanted into the trouble spots. Because of its origins, some patients are concerned about the risk of disease transmission, but this risk is minimal, thanks to the careful screening process that it undergoes. Finally, fascia doesn't seem to last longer than collagen.

Synthetic Fillers

SILICONE

Silicone is considered the black sheep of filler materials, a judgment that is not entirely unfair, considering its history of misuse. The biggest complaint about silicone has been that it tends to migrate from its intended location; another complaint was that many impure varieties of silicone were on the market.

The introduction of Silikon 1000, a silicone product approved by the FDA for the treatment of certain ophthalmologic conditions, has renewed interest in silicone fillers. Some physicians are using Silikon 1000 as an off-label cosmetic filler. Currently, its maker is in the process of implementing the trials necessary for the FDA's approval for cosmetic use.

If the procedures are done properly, the results with silicone can be excellent, but there are several crucial variables that determine a positive outcome. First, silicone must be injected slowly, with tiny droplets injected into the wrinkle at intervals separated by at least a month; therefore, deep wrinkles can take six months to a year to be fully corrected. As with other procedures that are classified as permanent, it's important to remember that nothing will keep further wrinkles from showing up. Bottom line: sooner or later, you'll need to return for a little fine-tuning.

Artecoll is a combination of bovine collagen and polymethyl-methacrylate, a Plexiglas-type sphere that can be injected into deep lines in the face and scars; it has been used in Canada, Europe, Mexico, and South America since 1993. The FDA studies have been submitted for evaluation, but as of the writing of this book, Artecoll is not yet available in the United States.

The collagen portion of Artecoll eventually disappears, but the sphere remains permanently. Some patients have seen great results with this filler, particularly in the treatment of wrinkles, but others have reported adverse reactions to the sphere, such as the development of lumps in the skin. It's also been noted that Artecoll can produce a bumpy effect in the lips. As Artecoll is mixed with bovine collagen, a skin test is required. The injection is administered similarly to collagen, except that some physicians like to tape the treated area for at least two days after the procedure so that the filler is able to settle into place.

My opinion on Artecoll is that if a patient is going to use a synthetic substance, it's a smarter idea to use a purely synthetic filler, such as silicone.

Implants

When filler implants were introduced almost thirty years ago, they offered great hope of being able to erase the ravages of time. In recent years, however, the initial excitement surrounding filler implants has definitely waned. High on the list of complaints is the tendency of implants to lose their original shape—they can get hard, contract, and even protrude from their original location. It is also difficult to ensure the right fit because implants—unlike injectable fillers—are linear and need to conform to a certain shape. Studies are also starting to find that implants can't be considered permanent. Aging, as we all know, is a continuous process, so what constitutes a major improvement today would be less of an improvement in a year's time. Also, even though an implant smooths certain creases really well, such as the nasolabial folds, it doesn't correct them entirely, making it necessary to have another filler injected over the implant for a complete correction.

Finally, in my experience I've found that patients want to improve their facial flaws quickly and effortlessly, and implants, because of the need for surgery and stitches, don't satisfy that desire.

HUMAN IMPLANTS: ALLODERM

Like Cymetra, Alloderm is derived from cadaver skin; but unlike Cymetra, which is an injectable, Alloderm comes in sheets and can be implanted in the skin for volume, as well as in the lips, by a minor surgical procedure. Alloderm has been used for a long time as a surface skin graft for treating burn patients. The result achieved with Alloderm was once thought to be permanent, but studies have found that after a year or less, most of the benefit will disappear.

SYNTHETIC IMPLANTS

Polytetrafluoroethylene, most commonly known as Gore-Tex, is a substance used for making swimsuits and ski jackets, and, more interestingly, for rejuvenating the face in the form of implants. Gore-Tex was created in the late 1960s for use in vascular surgery; today it is often used to correct deep nasolabial folds and other facial defects, and to augment the lips, often permanently. Unlike many other filler materials, polytetrafluoroethylene cannot be used to add volume to the face.

The implants are removable, should the patient decide to get rid of them. Another benefit is that since there is no risk of an allergic reaction, it is not necessary to spend time waiting for a skin test. Finding a physician who is properly trained and experienced in working with these implants, however, is crucial. Among the problems that could arise are migration of the material, an unnatural feel to the treated area, and skin infections.

- *Gore-Tex:* This threaded implant is guided into the dermis with a needle while the patient is under local anesthesia. In time, the patient's fibroblasts (the skin cells that make collagen) migrate into the implant and secure it in place.
- *UltraSoft Form:* This is the same substance, but in the form of small, pliable tubes. UltraSoft Form can be inserted into the skin to fill in deep lines on the face and to augment the lips.

As you can see, the options in filler materials are vast and constantly changing. Staying on top of breaking developments can be a full-time job! (And it is—mine.) While it's great to have so many options, it's crucial to remember that a wonderful outcome with a filler material is dependent not just on the material itself but also on the skill and expertise of the physician.

No matter how fantastic today's options, however, nothing stops the aging process. Aging is unavoidable and will happen to each and every one of us. The face is constantly changing, and a result that might look fantastic today will need tinkering with in the proverbial tomorrow. Continued maintenance is crucial, whether in a physician's office, at home with a solid skin care routine, or, better yet, both. Understand that concept and you're halfway there.

: The Right (Food) Stuff :

One of my best patients is a nutritionist with bustling practices in Miami and Ohio. On the basis of her professional and personal experience, she recommends a few simple nutrition guidelines both pre- and postprocedure. In her—and my—opinion, they can make the difference between a good result and a fantastic one.

- One week before, exclude: Aspirin, gingko biloba, garlic, coenzyme Q10, flax oil, cod liver oil, vitamin A, vitamin E, any other essential fatty acids
- 24 to 48 hours before, exclude: Niacin, high-sodium foods, high-sugar foods, refined carbohydrates (you may eat fruit; just avoid foods with added sugar, fructose, corn syrup, etc.), spicy foods, caffeine, alcohol, cigarettes
- 48 hours after your procedure you may begin adding: gingko biloba, garlic, coenzyme Q10, flax oil, cod liver oil, vitamin A, vitamin E, any other essential fatty acids
- 3 days to a week after your procedure, depending on your sensitivity level, you may add: higher-sodium foods, high-sugar foods, refined carbohydrates (you may eat fruit; just avoid foods with added sugar, fructose, corn syrup, etc.), caffeine, alcohol, cigarettes, flush-free niacin, aspirin, spicy foods

What can fillers do?

1. fill in lines
 a. smile lines (nasolabial folds)

b. lipstick (perioral) lines

c. marionette lines (oral commissures)

2. fill in scars

3. restore the contours of the lips

4. add fullness to the face, such as:

   a. cheeks

   b. cheekbones to restore youthful fullness

   c. lips

   d. chin

   e. temples

   f. under the eyes

What Botox does better

1. eliminate crow's feet

2. smooth specific lines

   a. forehead lines

   b. frown lines

   c. neck lines

   d. chest lines

: All Abroad :

The American market isn't the last word on filler materials—not that that's a bad thing. Step outside the United States, and the extensive list of fillers could boggle the mind of even the most informed patient. Thanks to our hypercautious safety practices, however, the majority of these fillers will probably never see the inside of your (American) physician's office. Remember, the fact that a filler is being used doesn't mean it's safe and free of risks.

Here, a brief overview.

AcHyal

Arteplast

Biocell Ultravital

Bioplastique

DermaLive

DermaDeep

Dermaplant

Endoplast-50

Evolution

fat autografting

Formacrill

Human Placental Collagen

Hyal-System

Hylan Rofilan Gel

Kopolymer

Meta-Crill

New-Fill

Permacol

Plasmagel

PMS 350

Profill

Resoplast

Reviderm Intra

Adatosil 5000

Silikon 1000

Surgisis

I think it's clear that collagen, which for years has been the gold standard of filler materials, is being challenged by some pretty serious competition, primarily from the Restylane group of materials. In fact, I think that of all the fillers currently available, Restylane is the one that is really going to shine in the years to come. Not only is it immensely versatile, both in its ability to restore youthful volume to the face and eliminate less-than-youthful lines and wrinkles, but it also lasts an incredibly long time and doesn't require a time-consuming skin test. That is a magical combination that I'm certain will leave patients happily, beautifully satisfied. Aside from a permanent antidote to aging, one couldn't ask for much more.

FILLERS AT A GLANCE

FILLER TYPE	FILLER NAME	SOURCE	WHAT DOES IT DO?	ALLERGY RISK?
Bovine Collagen	Zyderm I	bovine (cow)	smooths scars and superficial to moderately deep lines	YES
	Zyderm II	bovine (cow)	smooths scars and superficial to moderately deep lines	YES
	Zyplast	bovine (cow)	fills deeper wrinkles and furrows, nasolabial folds, deep scars; enhances lip border; plumps lips	YES
Human Collagen	Cosmoderm	infant foreskin cells	smooths scars and superficial to moderately deep lines on face	NO
	Cosmoplast	infant foreskin cells	fills deeper wrinkles and furrows, nasolabial folds, deep scars; enhances lip border; plumps lips	NO
Human Injectable Tissue	Cymetra	human cadaver skin	smooths scars and superficial to moderately deep lines	NO

cont.

FILLER TYPE	FILLER NAME	SOURCE	WHAT DOES IT DO?	ALLERGY RISK?
	Isolagen	fibroblasts from patient	produces collagen growth in skin	NO
Nonanimal Hyaluronic Acid	Restylane Fine Lines	hyaluronic acid equivalent engineered in a lab	smooths superficial lines	NO
	Restylane	hyaluronic acid equivalent engineered in a lab	smooths wrinkles; plumps lips and lip border	NO
	Perlane	hyaluronic acid equivalent engineered in a lab	smooths folds; volume augmentation (cheeks, chin, and lips)	NO
Animal-derived Hyaluronic Acid	Hylaform Fine Lines	rooster combs	smooths superficial lines	NO
	Hylaform	rooster combs	smooths wrinkles; plumps lips and lip border	NO
	Hylaform Plus	rooster combs	smooths folds; volume augmentation (cheeks, chin, and lips)	NO

FILLERS AT A GLANCE (*cont.*)

FILLER TYPE	FILLER NAME	SOURCE	WHAT DOES IT DO?	ALLERGY RISK?
Human	Fat	patient	smooths moderate to deep lines; volume augmentation (cheeks, chin, and lips)	NO
Human	Fascia	connective tissue of human cadavers	fills moderately deep lines	NO
Synthetic	Silicone	engineered in a lab	smooths fine to deep lines; volume augmentation (cheeks, chin, and lips)	NO
	Artecoll	Plexiglas-type sphere with bovine collagen	smooths moderate to deep lines; volume augmentation (cheeks, chin, and lips)	YES
Human Implants	Alloderm	cadaver skin	plumps lips and smooths deep lines	NO
Synthetic Implants	Gore-Tex	polytetrafluoroethylene	plumps lips and smooths deep lines	NO
	Ultrasoft Form	polytetrafluoroethylene	plumps lips and smooths deep lines	NO

six

: Radiance Revealed :

What is it about young, healthy skin that elicits a steady stream of compliments? An absence of lines and wrinkles might seem like the obvious answer, but actually, that doesn't paint the full picture. It turns out that radiance, which is hard to define but desired by everyone, is what signals to the world that all is well with your skin.

What is radiance? This nebulous expression is often used to describe those on the brink of a life-changing event, such as expectant mothers and blushing brides. Without a doubt, radiance is a term with connotations of happiness, health, and vitality. In a medical sense, a look of radiance can be attributed to a variety of elements. For starters, radiant skin is evenly pigmented, its texture is dewy and smooth, and the pores are so tiny that they might as well be invisible. The color of the skin, too, is alive and bright. Put it all together, and the end result is the kind of skin that looks beautiful even without a drop of makeup.

By now you're probably thinking that this dream skin is impossible to obtain and only babies and Hollywood starlets can claim it as their own. There is a certain element of truth to that statement, since the components of radiant skin—abundant collagen and elastin; minimal, if any, sun damage; and rapid cell turnover, to name just a few—come naturally to young people. Over time, however, these elements start to crumble. Even someone who has just turned thirty can have skin that doesn't replenish itself as quickly as it did a few years before, resulting in an accumulation of dead skin cells that contribute to how the skin reflects light. Throw in the lines and multiple brown spots that are usually the result of too much sun exposure, and it's easy to see why you now have a dull complexion of your very own.

Now, some good news: there are a multitude of cosmetic resurfacing procedures today to help you undo most, if not all, of this damage and ultimately reward you with a smooth, glowing complexion. As with every other goal related to flawless skin, being satisfied with your result goes hand in hand with an effective at-home skin care regimen. In an earlier chapter I explained how products containing alpha and beta hydroxy acids and retinol, to name just a few ingredients, are crucial because of their ability to thoroughly exfoliate the skin and possibly stir collagen production, in turn ensuring that your complexion will remain as smooth and even as possible. But as effective as these ingredients are in maintaining skin health and reversing some past damage, even they have their limitations. Need another solution? Enter the resurfacing treatment.

: What Is Skin Resurfacing? :

As the term implies, resurfacing treatments rid you of a mottled complexion and replace it with a much improved version.

This is accomplished in different ways and to varying degrees, but this much is true: if you don't like what Father Time has done to your skin, then by all means use a resurfacing treatment to improve on his work.

In this chapter I will be reviewing a range of procedures unsurpassed for attaining radiant skin. Some of these procedures, like light acid peels, rid the upper layer of the skin (stratum corneum) of accumulated dead skin cells and can be found at some spas as well as at the dermatologist's office. At the other end of the spectrum are the more invasive procedures, such as deep peels, dermabrasion, and certain lasers that actually penetrate past the stratum corneum and into the living tissues of the skin. There, the all-important collagen is stimulated and most pigmentation problems are taken care of. (This level of resurfacing should be entrusted only to a physician in a medical setting.) The deeper the treatment, the greater the result and, accordingly, the longer the recuperation.

Between these two extremes are a medley of treatments that deliver a significant enough change with a tolerable amount of discomfort. Certain types of lasers (including the new nonburning lasers) fall into this category, as do some chemical peels. Rounding out this group are microdermabrasion treatments.

Whatever your mission—from eradicating unpleasant reminders of your suntanning years to getting the radiant complexion you've always longed for—I'm pretty certain that you'll find answers here. The all-important question, of course, is which of these treatments is the appropriate one for you. This chapter, and your physician, will help you decide.

: Chemical Peels :

Chemical peels help improve many skin conditions, such as acne, melasma, uneven skin texture, brown spots, hyperpigmentation and wrinkling. Types of peeling are typically ranked as very superficial, superficial, medium, and deep; once the physician has assessed the condition of the skin, it is decided which of these four depths of peeling would be the most helpful. The lower-intensity peels tend to be very popular, particularly at spas and skin clinics, while medium and deep peels have declined in popularity, in large part because of the introduction of new laser procedures. Lasers can often yield the same results as deep peeling, if not better.

What Is in a Peel?

A lot of the same ingredients that are so effective in at-home care are used in much higher percentages in professional peels. They include the following:

GLYCOLIC ACID

The most common ingredient in chemical peels is glycolic acid, a star member of the alpha hydroxy group. As I explained in an earlier chapter, AHAs are derived from naturally occurring compounds, in this case sugarcane, and they work by inducing exfoliation and speeding the cell cycle. The typical concentration of a glycolic acid product tends to be no higher than 10 percent, while for a peel the concentration can climb up to 70 percent.

SALICYLIC ACID

The lone beta hydroxy acid, salicylic acid, is unrivaled in how well it treats acne-prone skin. For home use, most products have an average of 2 percent salicylic acid, while a typical concentration in a peel is 20 percent to 30 percent.

Resorcinol, a phenol derivative that can be used as an in-office peel either on its own or as a component of the popular peel called Jessner's solution, is used quite often. Jessner's solution, meanwhile, combines a hodgepodge of exfoliating ingredients, including resorcinol, salicylic acid, and lactic acid (also an AHA). It was developed by a dermatologist who wanted to reduce the concentration and toxicity of each of the individual ingredients while increasing overall efficacy. Another benefit of Jessner's solution is that it can be layered under other peels for even more dramatic improvement.

Trichloroacetic acid (TCA) is usually reserved for superficial and medium-depth peels. If administered often enough, a low-concentration (usually 10 percent to 15 percent) TCA peel can remove fine wrinkles and leave the skin with a smooth finish. Once the intensity is increased to the standard 35 percent, it is able to delve deeper, but with a longer recuperation time.

The most invasive peel is done with phenol and can improve the complexion dramatically. It has many disadvantages, however; and as I mentioned earlier, lasers have pretty much taken over where deep peels left off.

With every resurfacing technique mentioned here, I insist that you entrust your face to only the most experienced physician. Many variables can affect the outcome of a chemical peel, most of which aren't readily apparent. In other words, in the hands of different physicians the same ingredient will deliver a different outcome.

The most basic factor is what type of acid is used and in what percentage, and in some cases the pH level. The higher the pH, the more basic the solution; the lower the pH, the more acidic. Other considerations are the technique used in applying the solution. Is it being painted on lightly or rubbed in? How long is it being kept on the skin? How does the physician prepare the skin before the peel? What skin care regimen is the patient following? Does it include a product with highly active ingredients, like Retin-A? What kind of skin does the patient have? Is she an Italian woman with thick, oily skin? Or is she a blonde who's had a face-lift and thinned skin to show for it? The attention paid to these variables is monumentally important in determining a successful outcome.

Just like the face, the hands, neck, and chest are often exposed to the sun and receive their share of damage. But unlike the face, which responds extremely well to stronger peels—thanks to its rich supply of oil glands—other areas of the body can't be peeled as deeply without risking scars.

Very Superficial Peels

Just about everybody can benefit from a very superficial peel, from younger patients with minimal imperfections to older patients who haven't exposed their skin to a lot of sun. The number one benefit of a very superficial peel is its effectiveness at removing the dead skin cells that stubbornly cling to the skin's outer layer, the stratum corneum, in the process yielding skin that is smoother in texture and more evenly pigmented. Those with acne can see a great improvement, such as in the cleansing of blocked pores and the fading of any leftover dark marks. A patient can also expect the removal of freckles, certain types of melasma, and solar lentigos (sun spots). Fine wrinkles can be improved considerably, but a very superficial peel does very little for deeper lines. After several treatments, the repetitive peeling action, or exfoliation, can stimulate growth of the epidermis and even lead to regeneration of collagen.

A bit of patience always comes in handy, and it will be put to good use in this instance. Basically, when the peeling is this superficial, it's unrealistic to expect a whole new you after just one treatment. It usually takes at least four peels, spaced approximately three weeks apart, before you can begin to see an improvement.

Suggested Peels

- glycolic acid at 30 percent to 50 percent (depending on the pH factor)
- Jessner's solution
- TCA (10 percent to 15 percent)

Recuperation

None. You might be a little pink, but it's nothing that a touch of makeup can't disguise.

Suggested Frequency

Initially: every three to four weeks
Maintenance: every two months

Superficial Peels

Slightly stronger than very superficial peels, superficial peels penetrate deeper into the epidermis and are ideal for those with even more sun damage and other texture imperfections.

Suggested Treatments

- glycolic acid at 50 percent to 70 percent (depending on the pH factor)

- resorcinol at 40 percent to 50 percent
- TCA at 20 percent

Similar to recuperation with a very superficial peel, but with additional peeling and flaking of the skin. These effects can last up to a week and in some cases resemble a light sunburn.

Initially: every four weeks
Maintenance: three months

Medium Peels

Now we're getting somewhere! Medium-depth peels go past the epidermis and affect the upper portion of the dermis, which is where the blood vessels and the collagen reside. This process of inflaming the skin helps to produce new collagen. Essentially, anytime that the collagen is manipulated it results in a firming action and, later down the road, an increase in natural collagen.

This level of peeling is great for someone with moderate wrinkling and acne. Deep lines will be softened, although not entirely eliminated, while nearly all brown spots will be erased.

One caveat is that medium-depth peels are generally appropriate only for skin types I through III, as classified by the Fitzpatrick Skin Type system. (Refer to Chapter 2 for more information on these classifications.) Darker skin tones, such as those in types IV to VI, can benefit from a medium peel. But if the peel is done improperly, there is a greater risk of developing postinflammatory hyperpigmentation.

- glycolic acid at 70 percent (depends on the pH factor)
- TCA at 35 percent
- Augmented TCA Plus: glycolic acid at 70 percent plus TCA at 35 percent
- Carbon Dioxide Flush plus TCA at 35 percent

RECUPERATION

Expect to look pretty bad for the first ten days following a medium-depth peel. On days one and two the skin appears slightly pink. On days three and four, the skin darkens. By day five the skin begins to peel off. Finally, by day ten the peeling should be completed and you'll be able to flaunt your newly rejuvenated self.

SUGGESTED FREQUENCY

Once a year, if needed.

Deep Peels

Deep peels are turning into the endangered species of the resurfacing world, and anyone familiar with how they work will understand why. This level of peeling is done with phenol, an acid that has the ability to penetrate down to the deepest levels of the skin. For the procedure, the patient is sedated and hooked up to a cardiac monitor, and his or her vital signs are repeatedly checked for irregularities. The recuperation time is also lengthy—the skin is raw for two or three weeks and remains pink for two to three months. Other risks include a possible loss of pigmentation, called hypopigmentation, resulting in a face that is much lighter than the neck and body.

On the upside, since the peel is penetrating the skin more deeply, it produces long-lasting and extremely dramatic improvement. By reaching deep into the collagen layer, the skin is able to regenerate more of it. The ideal patient would be one with severe sun damage, such as crosshatch lines on the cheeks and leathery skin.

SUGGESTED TREATMENT

- phenol peel

RECUPERATION

There's no elegant way to word this. After a deep peel the skin is in pretty bad shape for two weeks, and pink for months.

SUGGESTED FREQUENCY

Once in a lifetime.

⋮ Laser (Light Amplification by the Stimulated Emission of Radiation) ⋮

When the buzz on lasers as an antiaging tool first started in the early 1990s, people didn't know what to make of it. To most people, lasers were symbols of the kind of high-tech wizardry associated with the characters in *Star Wars*. Faster than the speed of light, however, lasers went from being a novel idea of the future to a much-improved alternative to the cosmetic procedures that already existed.

Almost five years later, laser technology has evolved into a mighty presence in cosmetic improvements. In the past, lasers were limited to the treatment of certain cosmetic conditions, such as birthmarks, that affected only a small group of people.

That all changed with the introduction of the carbon dioxide (CO_2) laser, the first of its kind to actually resurface the skin. Before the CO_2 laser, the only other procedure that could regenerate the superficial and deep layers of skin were a deep phenol peel and dermabrasion. Not long afterward, it seemed as if new cosmetic lasers were being introduced every day.

A lot of my patients tell me that they're afraid of lasers—usually because they assume that there's only one type of (scary) laser—but I reassure them that "lasers" is just an umbrella term encompassing different treatments. I liken this situation to airplanes and cars, which are different forms of transportation with similar engineering characteristics.

Lasers work by aiming a beam of amplified light at the skin; when the beam hits the skin, it is attracted to certain components. For example, a laser for brown spots is attracted to melanin, or pigment, and a vascular laser is attracted to the red blood vessels. Since the subject of lasers is vast enough to fill an entire book, we will limit our discussion to the cosmetic lasers that are indispensable for bringing out your beauty.

What are lasers used for?

- port wine stains and birthmarks
- wrinkles and lines
- superficial brown spots
- deep pigmented spots
- scars and stretch marks
- broken blood vessels
- warts
- hair removal
- tattoo removal

Ablative Lasers

CARBON DIOXIDE (CO_2) LASER

Almost a decade ago, people who were contemplating "getting a little something done" were drawn to lasers, which promised to bust wrinkles and, overall, rejuvenate the skin. At the time, the carbon dioxide (CO_2) resurfacing laser, which is still around today, was being touted as a one-stop solution for various conditions, especially severely sun-damaged skin. This laser delivers results comparable to those from a deep phenol peel, minus the risks to health. It is also one example of ablative (or burning) lasers, which work by heating the surface of the skin in order to penetrate into the deepest layers. In the case of the CO_2 laser, an amplified wavelength of light is directed at the skin and is immediately attracted to the water in the skin. The water absorbs the light, in the process removing years of sun spots, wrinkles, and other remnants of accumulated damage. The patient's skin is red and swollen immediately following the treatment, with full recovery coming slowly after two weeks, when new skin has grown in.

If this process sounds serious, that's because it is very serious—a fact that at the time wasn't emphasized nearly enough. Not only is the recovery long and often painful, but there can be serious side effects, such as scarring and loss of pigment. Also, people mistakenly thought that they would never get another wrinkle, which is a nice idea but, as we all know, definitely untrue. Today, some patients still underestimate the power of this laser and request it in order to treat a few lines. I reply that this would be like using a cannon to kill a fly.

I think that although CO_2 lasers are great for certain people, they were initially overused. Someone with a few lines doesn't need to be resurfaced. Often, a filler like collagen could be injected instead to alleviate the problem. CO_2 lasers are also not for someone with dynamic wrinkles around the eyes. Botox is better suited to treat such wrinkles, which will only come back. As with any other procedure, the usefulness of a CO_2 laser has to be determined on a person-by-person basis. It's not a magic wand.

Recuperation

Two weeks of no makeup, with the skin remaining pink for two to three months.

Suggested Frequency

Once or twice in a lifetime

ERBIUM:YAG LASER

Less dramatic in effect than the CO_2 laser, but nonetheless very effective at improving wrinkles, the Erbium:YAG was, and still is today, a moderate alternative to the CO_2 laser. The skin isn't heated as much with this laser, but you won't get as deep or dramatic a result, either. It's great for people with mild to moderate sun damage. The Erbium is comparable to a medium-depth peel.

Recuperation

It'll be a week before you can wear makeup, and you'll experience a month of redness.

Suggested Frequency

Once every five years, if necessary.

Pigment Lasers

If someone could play "connect the dots" with the brown spots on your hands, face, shoulders, and chest, then you're a candidate for a treatment with a pigment laser. These spots, typically referred to as "liver spots," are caused by irregular production of melanin brought on by—what else?—the sun. The specific pigment in the laser acts as a magnet, drawing the light only to the pigment while sparing the surrounding skin.

COMMON PIGMENT LASERS

Q-switched ruby
Q-switched alexandrite
Q-switched Nd:YAG
Aura

RECUPERATION

Immediately after the treatment, the skin will be red and scabs will start to form. In about a week the facial skin will be sufficiently healed so that you can wear makeup. The hands take about two weeks to heal, the arms three weeks, and the legs almost a month. All areas will have some redness for several months afterward.

SUGGESTED FREQUENCY

One session is usually sufficient to remove all visible spotting. But remember, inadequate sun protection will lead to a slew of new spots.

Vascular Lasers

A certain degree of rosiness is always desirable, but not when it's in the form of severe redness on the face, most prominently on the cheeks and around the corners of the nose. This is usually a direct result of dilated or broken blood vessels. Vascular lasers can help. Rosacea, a chronic condition that brings about a lot of involuntary blushing, also benefits from such lasers. Finally, most types of red birthmarks can be eradicated quickly with this treatment.

In this instance, the laser targets the hemoglobin (red pigment in the bloodstream) that lies within the vessels.

COMMON VASCULAR LASERS

VersaPulse
Aura
Vbeam

RECUPERATION

The skin bounces back almost immediately afterward.

SUGGESTED FREQUENCY

As needed.

Nonablative (Nonburning) Laser Resurfacing

One of the most innovative of nonsurgical cosmetic treatments, nonablative laser resurfacing is the perfect solution for those who want to improve their complexions at their own pace. The term "ablative" refers to the act of removing the surface of the skin. (I know it's hard to imagine this, since there's not a scalpel in sight!) The nonablative treatments, meanwhile, rejuvenate the skin without creating a wound that needs time to heal.

Not surprisingly, one session of a nonablative treatment won't deliver the same dramatic result as a CO_2 laser. Actually, a series of four to six treatments will be required before the patient sees a change. On the upside, the recuperation time is nil.

RECUPERATION

None whatsoever. You can hop onto the exam table and hop right off.

SUGGESTED FREQUENCY

Four to six treatments are required.

COMMON NONABLATIVE LASERS

CoolTouch
SmoothBeam
N-Lite
Aura and Lyra laser combination

: Intense Pulsed Light (IPL) :

IPL is usually mentioned in the same breath as laser treatments, but unlike lasers, which amplify one wavelength of light, IPL treatments use a multitude of wavelengths, depending on the desired results. The ideal conditions for this treatment are hyperpigmentation, freckles, ruddiness, broken blood vessels, early sun spots, large pores, fine lines, and lax skin.

IPL Facial
FotoFacial
PhotoFacial
Photorejuvenation
EpiFacial

RECUPERATION

This is a true "lunchtime" procedure, with no recuperation time whatsoever.

SUGGESTED FREQUENCY

Once a month for four months.

: Coblation (Electrosurgical Cold Ablation) :

Coblation delivers to the skin a saline solution through which a cool electric current is passed. A subsequent reaction specifically heats and vaporizes the top layer of skin. Known as Visage, this technique is very effective for mild to moderate wrinkles and sun damage in people with all skin types.

RECUPERATION

The skin will be tender for five to seven days. Overall redness will subside in a month.

SUGGESTED FREQUENCY

Once every five years, if necessary.

: Mechanical Exfoliation :

Dermabrasion

Dermabrasion is still popular with physicians who have experience in it. Experience is crucial, since this procedure is truly an inexact science. A rapidly rotating wheel studded with diamond particles deeply abrades the skin and causes it to bleed and crust. When the procedure is done correctly, though, the results are fantastic.

RECUPERATION

It'll be a week to ten days before you can wear makeup, and several months before the redness subsides.

SUGGESTED FREQUENCY

Can be done once or twice in a lifetime.

MICRODERMABRASION

There are certain people who adore the idea of scrubbing away all imperfections, and those folks will probably love microdermabrasion. This treatment, which is helpful for improving skin texture, unblocking pores, removing excess oil, and possibly reducing wrinkles, works in the following way: As the small microdermabrasion machine bombards the skin with thousands of sterilized aluminum oxide crystals, a vacuum suction removes these particles along with the dislodged skin. The force at which the particles are propelled and the speed at which the device is passed over the skin determine the depth of the treatment. There is a small risk of certain side effects, such as bleeding, infection, and hyperpigmentation; but overall, I think that microdermabrasion can be useful and safe if done by a properly trained physician. It's also a technique that can be overused, so I'd advise that it be done no more than twelve to twenty times a year.

The most common particle used is the aluminum oxide crystal, but since the introduction of microdermabrasion just a few years ago, other particles, like salt crystals, are making headlines. There are also more microdermabrasion treatments on the market than there are wrinkles on the face, but essentially they all perform the same function. Microdermabrasion is equivalent to having a light acid peel.

RECUPERATION

Aside from minor pinkness, there are no adverse effects.

SUGGESTED FREQUENCY

No more than twelve to twenty times a year.

TYPICAL MICRODERMABRASION TREATMENTS

Dermapeel
Power Peel
Parisian Peel
Diamond Peel
Silk Peel

There are many ways to get to your desired end point, and which route to take should be a joint decision by you and your physician. Again, I must stress how important it is to stay out of the sun. Why undergo another procedure when a few simple precautionary steps can keep you beautiful for a long, long time? Point taken? Good.

seven

: Befores and Afters :

I t's been said that pictures speak louder than words, and this is never truer than when the topic is the transformative powers of today's nonsurgical cosmetic procedures. One of my missions in this book has been to provide you with the basic facts regarding these procedures, and while I hope I've met that goal, I understand that words can only say so much. Without a doubt, it's one thing for you to read all about these new techniques and quite another to actually see them put to the test.

And have we put them to the test! Read on as Andrea, Linda, Maija, and Brenda, our four female volunteers—who range in age from thirty-nine to fifty-four years old—candidly describe the specific ways that aging is affecting their looks. Their motivations for submitting their faces to any combination of today's hottest cosmetic procedures—Botox, collagen, and Restylane injections—are quite typical, and as stunning as the series of before and after pictures are, I'm happy to report that the results are also typical.

Andrea Cantor, Thirty-Nine Years Old
Treated with: Botox

Dr. Brandt's View

Even though her life was consumed with raising her three young daughters and co-running a successful publicity firm in Westchester, New York, Andrea Cantor never forgot that a very significant birthday, the big four-oh, was almost upon her. It didn't make a difference when her friends assured her repeatedly that she looked very youthful (which she does); Andrea was adamant about greeting this occasion with a little beautification.

On the day of her appointment, I studied Andrea carefully, paying special attention to her facial expressions. Immediately, I noticed that her face was very animated and always lit up in a huge smile. Ordinarily, I'm not against such vigor and vitality, but in a cosmetic sense, it's this type of abundant dynamic movement that is responsible for those first signs of wrinkling. I also noticed that like a lot of women her age, Andrea was starting to have an accumulation of loose tissue under her eyes and a slight bulge right underneath her eyelids that became very apparent when she smiled. Most patients mistake this bulge for excess fat, when in fact it's an overworked muscle that can benefit from a treatment like Botox. Right above her eyes, I noted a few lines on her forehead; and lower on the face, Andrea had the beginnings of jowl formation and her jawline was starting to lose definition.

I realize that this sounds like a lengthy list of conditions to treat, especially in only one visit, but since most of Andrea's "faults" were related to muscle activity, I decided to treat her with Botox, which is supereffective for this form of wrinkling. Also, I felt that for someone like Andrea, who had never had a cosmetic procedure and who didn't need plastic surgery just yet, Botox would be the ideal starter procedure. I began by injecting her forehead lines, but I intentionally left some lines intact because otherwise I risked giving her a frozen expression and a lowered brow. Instead, the combination of moderately treating her forehead and injecting over her eyebrows left Andrea with a beautifully open and alert look.

Since the bulge under her eyes is due to muscular contractions, I treated her there, too, and this beautifully opened up her lower eyelid area without a need for surgery. Last, I gave her a few shots in her neck, and almost immediately we both saw her neck tighten up and her jowls become less apparent.

I think Andrea will be welcoming her fortieth birthday beautifully!

HOMECARE PRESCRIPTION

- v-zone neck cream will maintain firmness and elasticity in the neck area as well as smooth skin texture
- lineless eye cream to reduce puffiness and dark circles, promote firmness, and smooth signs of aging

Andrea's View

I am about to turn forty—ouch!—and I told my husband that for my birthday I wanted a little lift and softness around my eyes, mainly so that I wouldn't always look so tired. To me, the wrinkles that were beginning to develop on my forehead and the vertical line by my brows were screaming "forty, forty, forty!" That vertical line also made my eyes look droopy and tired.

I also said I'd consider a tummy tuck, but I would never

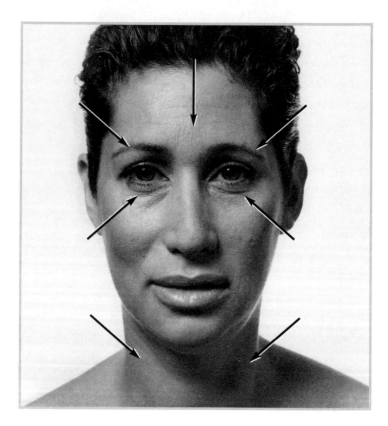

Andrea Cantor, Before

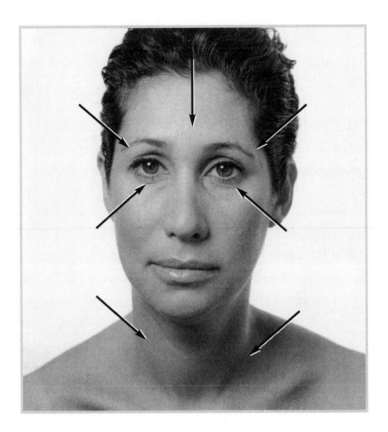

Andrea Cantor, After

really go through with it and I figured the cosmetic treatment would be more realistic. I guess I was looking for the instant shot (no pun intended!) of gratification that Botox can deliver. To me, a Botox injection is no different from any other grooming technique, like coloring my hair, that will instantly make me look better. For almost a year now, I had been contemplating having Botox, and the desire has only grown stronger. In fact, I had just started to look into making an appointment with a dermatologist when this opportunity arose.

I was very excited about the procedure, not really nervous at all, and I was particularly looking forward to meeting the famous Dr. Brandt; I've heard and read so much about him. He has so much experience with Botox, and if anyone was qualified to shoot me up, I felt that he was definitely the one. My only fear was that my facial expressions would look forced. Plastic surgery never truly entered my mind, because I've seen a lot of bad plastic surgery and I thought I was too young for that, anyway. Maybe my feelings will change as I get older, but I find the idea of going under the knife very unnerving. I'm hoping that genetics, a good skin care regimen, and proper sun protection will go a long way.

On the day of the treatment, I opted to have the numbing cream applied to my face for approximately thirty minutes beforehand. I'm sure that helped, because the procedure was pretty painless, with the exception of the area between my brows—and at worst that felt like a pinch. The nurse had warned me that since this particular area has the thickest muscle, it might feel a bit uncomfortable. The only other slightly freaky part was when he injected my lower eyelid. I was not expecting that—I didn't even know that that area could be treated with Botox—and it was frightening to see a needle coming toward my eye!

At one point, Dr. Brandt said that he was going to treat my neck and I thought he was joking—did I have any wrinkles there? But before long I was making all the clenching motions he requested. The injections there were absolutely painless—it was hard to believe he was truly treating my neck.

Overall, I am quite pleased with the results, since they are very subtle and natural-looking. Other than my husband and a few of my friends, no one knows that I've had this done. I am getting all kinds of compliments, though, on how great my skin is looking. The areas around my eyes are definitely softer, and my eyes look so open and bright, but I am not quite sure that I see a difference in the horizontal lines by my brows. I would most definitely go back for more treatments. It was a great experience and I would tell others that it's a fast, mostly painless way to get an instant boost.

Linda Asch, Fifty Years Old
Treated with: Botox

Dr. Brandt's View

There are many reasons why people decide to enhance their appearance. In the case of Linda Asch, the decision truly had a higher meaning. Her beloved husband of barely a year had succumbed to cancer just a few months earlier, and during his illness Linda never had the time, or the inclination, to take a good look in the mirror. In her grief, she even stopped taking yoga classes, which used to bring her such great joy.

When I met Linda, she told me that she'd had silicone injected into her smile lines, as well as Botox, years earlier. The silicone, a permanent filler, was still in place, but naturally, any remnants of the Botox were long gone. I was struck by how beautiful Linda's skin was, but nevertheless, I made mental notes of the areas that could be improved. They included her eyes, which were slightly drooping, loose skin in

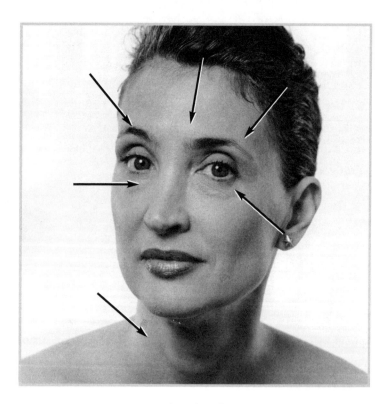

Linda Asch, Before

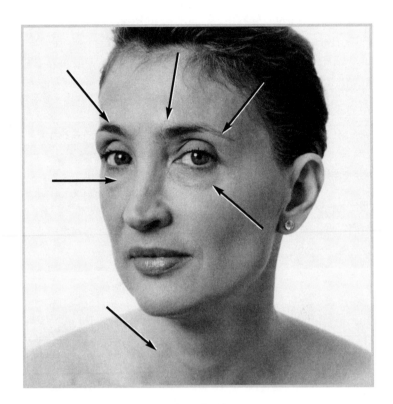

Linda Asch, After

her neck, and the jowls that were beginning to form along her jawline. Luckily for Linda, these are the areas that Botox is unrivaled at treating, so I used it everywhere: on her neck to eliminate the lines there and create nice definition in her jawline; around her eyes to open them up; on her brows; a touch on the moderately deep lines on her forehead; and even in the chin, since she was showing signs of dimpling in that area.

You'll be the judge, but I think that Linda now looks as beautiful on the outside as she is on the inside.

HOMECARE PRESCRIPTION

- "c" gel will firm and restore radiance to the skin, reducing free-radicals induced by stress
- "a" cream night to rejuvenate the appearance of tired skin, smooth away fine lines and wrinkles as well as stimulate collagen

Linda's View

Turning fifty years old wasn't such a big deal for me. I've always been very physically active, so I was never really beauty-conscious as much as I was body-conscious. I spent six months taking care of my sick husband, and there came a point when I couldn't do yoga anymore. Actually, I couldn't really leave the house to follow any kind of normal routine.

After he died, I took the first long look at myself in the mirror, and I felt as though I had aged. I'd been participating in a bereavement group for a while, and at some point I thought that it would be nice to treat myself to a rejuvenating procedure.

Four years ago, I had had Botox on my frown lines, and I was looking forward to doing it again. I had once thought that I could grow old gracefully, but now I hope to grow old gracefully with nonsurgical procedures! I think it's all a mind-set. I think that Jessica Tandy's wrinkled face was beautiful. I also loved Gloria Steinem's reply to someone who told her she looked good for someone who was fifty: "This is what fifty looks like." I feel the same way, and I hope to feel this way when I turn sixty.

I know that Botox isn't really botulism, so I don't really worry about it too much. It was pretty funny to see Dr. Brandt's nurse come into the exam room with a bucket of needles, but I guess it was all worth it, since none of my friends have told me, "Oh, you've had Botox!" Instead, they comment on how well rested I look. After the year I've had, I take that as a great compliment.

Maija Arbolino, Thirty-Nine Years Old
Treated with: Botox, Collagen, and Restylane

Dr. Brandt's View

Between her constant travels around the world for her career as a director of finance for a nonprofit organization in Manhattan, and zipping around with her energetic toddler, Maija has been too preoccupied with life to do much more about her appearance than basic maintenance. At almost forty, Maija is still a young woman, but she's already exhibiting a lot of the facial changes that you would see in a fair-skinned person who's had a lot of sun exposure. She needed total face rejuvenation, and using techniques like Botox, collagen, and Perlane, a form of Restylane that is sure to be the next hot cosmetic treatment, allowed me to restore her youthful appearance by filling instead of pulling the skin as a face-lift would have done. By comparison, a face-lift would remove any extra skin in her neck, but it would only make her face narrower and do little else for her overall appearance.

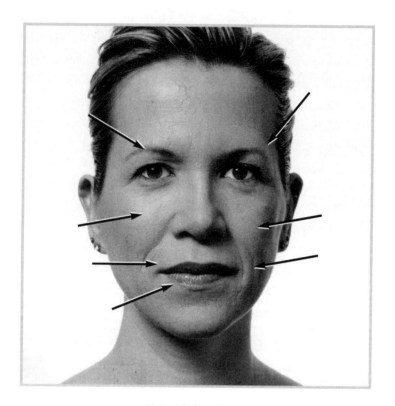

Maija Arbolino, Before

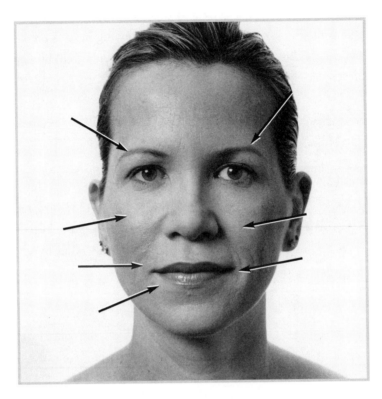

Maija Arbolino, After

I also decided to use Botox on her forehead, between the brows, on the neck—basically, everywhere. For her prominent nasolabial creases and marionette lines, I opted to use collagen, which required Maija to have two allergy tests, spaced two weeks apart, to ensure that she wouldn't have a bad reaction to it. I also treated the borders of her lips with collagen, which would eliminate any annoying lipstick bleeding. Last, I thought that Perlane would be great at building up her cheekbones, in the process adding a flattering contour to her face.

In my opinion, Maija's "after" picture could easily be a picture of herself from when she was in her twenties!

HOMECARE PRESCRIPTION

- "c" cream will address dehydration and discoloration due to sun exposure and minimize fine lines and wrinkles
- lightening gel fades sun and age spots as well as hyperpigmentation quickly and efficiently

Maija's View

I had a horrifying realization the other day. Not only was I about to turn forty, but I look it! All my life I've always looked younger than my age, but I feel that aging somehow sneaked up on me. What used to be cute dimples on my cheeks have turned into deep creases. I was also becoming obsessed with my other creases, both around my eyes and on my forehead. And where did this weird crepiness come from? I've seen other women my age whose skin looks way better. I'm sure it's from my years of being out in the sun and of thinking that I was indestructible. I've always thought I looked better with a tan—I still think I look better with a tan—but I now believe self-tanners are the only way to go.

I had been thinking that maybe it was time to get a little

something done, but I wanted it to be something that didn't include going under the knife. I've seen some really good face-lifts so I know it's possible to have great results, but if you can tell you've had a lift, then that's not a good thing. Just look at the society pages in the *Times*! Also, I figured that with surgery you could get a blood clot and die from your face-lift. Wouldn't that be a really stupid way to die?

The possibility of Botox was already in my radar because I had been hearing a lot about it and, actually, the fact that it was a form of botulism didn't scare me. I like the fact that Botox is temporary, and besides, I hadn't heard about anyone dropping dead from it.

It was so hectic in Dr. Brandt's office that first day of my treatments. I had already gotten over my initial apprehension and concern about what I was going to look like, which was good, considering that I've never even had a facial. Finally, Dr. Brandt breezed in with these wild lab glasses on his face, said hello, and started to scope my face. He was very to the point but also very entertaining. It's like he's the rock star of the dermatology world. I didn't think the Botox was very painful at all, and on my neck it was literally painless. On my car ride home, I had to make all these crazy faces—repeatedly frowning and smiling—to make sure that the Botox adhered properly. A few days later, it must have kicked in because I really noticed a difference. The crease between my eyebrows (which I affectionately call the "11") really disappeared, my forehead was smoothed out, and the crow's feet were completely gone.

I had never been treated with collagen before, so I had to wait for the two collagen tests that I had had at Dr. Brandt's office to come back. When I was finally deemed ready, I returned for more treatments. On that second visit, Dr. Brandt injected my smile lines and the "commas" around my mouth with collagen and with Restylane (which didn't need a test) around my cheekbones. Those injections were less painful than Botox, kind of like tweezings.

Now, I think that I finally look as if I've gotten all my sleep. With the results that I got, I would seriously consider doing it all again. I'm already dreading the day that it all disappears; I really don't want those creases back. My identical twin sister is also carefully watching me, and I think she's using me as a guinea pig before having anything done to herself. These treatments have also really come in handy at work, particularly when people tell me things that I find completely ridiculous. I have a better poker face now.

Brenda Segel, Fifty-Four Years Old
Treated with: Botox and Restylane

Dr. Brandt's View

There's something about significant birthdays that steers people into giving in to that ever-growing desire to have "something done." Brenda, a vice president at a book publishing company in Manhattan, grew up hearing her mother's (well-intentioned) insistence that she have her nose "fixed," starting when Brenda graduated from high school. Unwilling to give in to societal pressure to look a certain way, Brenda didn't change her nose until a monumental birthday, her fortieth, landed her in a plastic surgeon's office for that long-anticipated nose job. (While there, Brenda went ahead and had her eyes done, too.)

Almost fifteen years later, the temptation to tinker with her looks surfaced again, and this time Brenda opted to go with Botox and collagen injections.

When I first met Brenda, I noticed that her skin was starting to take on the characteristics usually seen in women in their fifties; her jawline was sagging, and her cheeks appeared deflated. She also had a bit of wrinkling around her eyes and on her forehead. For these reasons, I felt that Brenda was a perfect candidate for Perlane, and Brenda was intrigued to hear that I was going to treat her with this version of Restylane instead of with collagen; she loved the idea that this was the most durable material available today.

Of course, I also used quite a bit of Botox on her, but I didn't concentrate it in one specific area. Thanks to the versatility of Botox, I was able to use it throughout her entire face including her neck, both for the sagging there and to alleviate the jowling, on her crow's feet, under the eyes, and on the brows to give her a beautiful lift (a.k.a. the Botox face-lift).

I think Brenda looks amazing.

HOMECARE PRESCRIPTION

- lineless cream to restore a healthy glow to the skin while minimizing fine lines and wrinkles
- "c" eye cream to firm the eye contour, maintaining optimal hydration and smoothing signs of aging

Brenda's View

I might not be one of those people who are forever looking in the mirror, but I do feel better if I think I look better, be it through a good haircut, a nice new outfit, or Botox. We live in a time when people are living longer. Most of us baby boomers don't feel that we are the age that we really are, so we're often shocked when we see pictures of ourselves. For me, it was partly hearing people tell me that I looked tired and partly looking in the mirror and not only seeing wrinkles but feeling that the lower half of my face was falling in on itself. I also felt that my mouth and smile were starting to look crooked. I did not feel like having major surgery, so when the opportunity to work with Dr. Brandt in a completely noninvasive way presented itself, I jumped at it. And the way that I see it, if it's

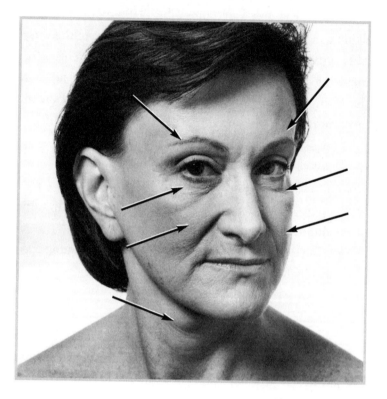

Brenda Segel, Before

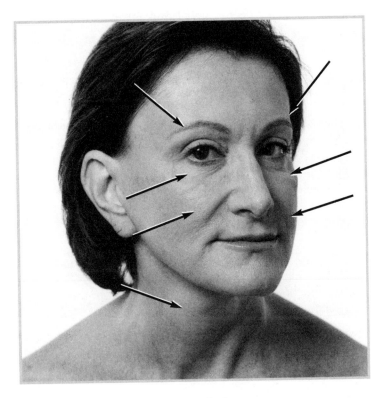

Brenda Segel, After

possible to improve your appearance quite safely, and if it makes you feel better about yourself, why not do it? Isn't that the whole point?

I was very excited about meeting Dr. Brandt, since his reputation is so stellar. I've had both Botox and collagen before, by more than one doctor, and I must say I now realize that technique is everything. While all my previous treatments showed results, none were as striking as those by Dr. Brandt. He injects Botox not just between the eyes, but above the brows, too. It's like having a brow-lift, and all of a sudden your eyes are slightly larger and people start telling you how good you look. Also, with him, the Botox injections hardly hurt at all—and that was without any numbing cream.

The Perlane was a bit more painful, but tolerable. I was numbed with cream for about twenty minutes before the procedure, and when it was time for the big moment, he injected me everywhere! He treated my cheeks, the frown lines from my nose to the corners of my mouth, the corners of my mouth, and the fine lines around my lips. Oddly enough, the first time I met Dr. Brandt he told me he wanted to do "something about those lips." I was a little nervous, since I fear looking like certain celebrities with overdone lips who shall remain nameless, but I was nonetheless excited to entrust my face to him. There was some stinging and burning afterward, but the cool gel pads that were placed on my skin did the trick. During the injections there is some bleeding and some redness afterward, so since I was going out to dinner with a friend, I definitely had to use makeup to cover up. My friend didn't mention my appearance, but when I told him what I'd just experienced, he told me that I looked terrific.

Years ago, I had collagen injections to soften the lines that ran from my nose to the corners of my mouth, but the change was so subtle that it hardly seemed worth all the effort. Dr. Brandt's technique was very interesting and obviously effective. First, he injected the Perlane into my cheeks, which lifted my skin and made the lines less prevalent and heavy. He then injected these lines, and the result was instantly dramatic. Again, technique was everything. I know that people are having Botox parties all over America, but truly, the right doctor makes all the difference.

As for plastic surgery, I'm not opposed to having it someday, since I think that lots of great things are being done these days, but it doesn't fill my heart with joy to think of the anesthesia and the recovery time that come along with it.

The doctor worked quickly and expertly, and he always made sure to ask me how I was holding up. He really is delightful and obviously passionate about what he does. I got the sense that Dr. Brandt is a real artist and his work, for him, is a labor of love. The results have more than met my expectations, and I would definitely consider doing it again, probably as a touch-up here and there after a few months have passed.

: Glamour Gals :

From a purely clinical point of view, the results obtained by our four volunteers were instantaneous and dramatic. But, we wondered, just how rejuvenated would our volunteers look once they weren't posed just so? Judging by these pictures— hair flowing, smiles shining brightly—aging has never looked so good.

For a full listing of dr. brandt homecare products, please see the Appendix.

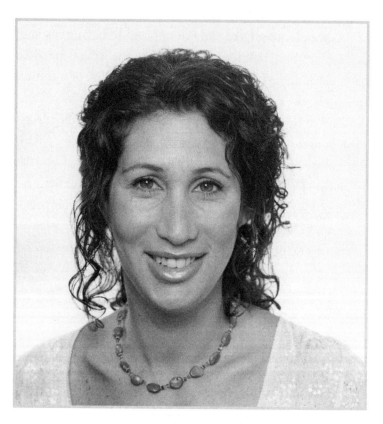

Andrea Cantor

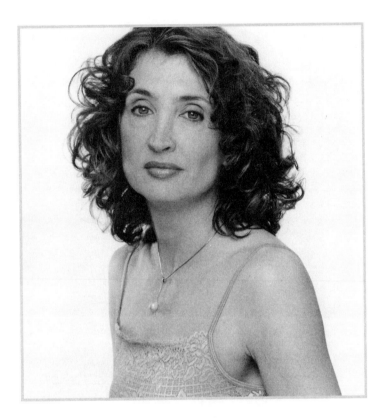

Linda Asch

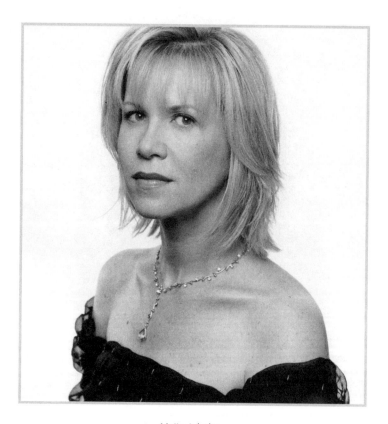

Maija Arbolino

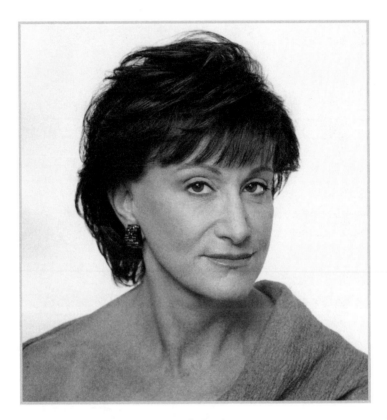

Brenda Segel

APPENDIX

Throughout this book, I've described in detail the many wonderful benefits that can be derived from a comprehensive skin care regimen, one that is chock-full of protective antioxidants, nurturing botanicals, and a fair sprinkling of active dermatological ingredients. When I created my own skin care collection, called simply "dr. brandt," almost three years ago, my motivation was multifold. First, my many patients were demanding it. I was constantly doling out product recommendations, and while I felt that there were many good product lines available, there really wasn't one line that had all the attributes I considered essential for flawless skin.

Second, and perhaps most important, during my medical internship at Memorial Sloan-Kettering Cancer Center in New York, I got to learn a great deal about the anticancer properties that other cultures, such as Asian cultures, were obtaining through their diet. It's no secret that these cultures suffer less drastically from certain ailments that plague Americans, such as obesity and cancer. It's been proved that the good health enjoyed by Asian cultures can be directly attributed to a diet rich in antioxidant ingredients like fish and green tea. In China and Japan, for example, people customarily drink four (or more) cups of tea daily.

As the possibility of creating my own skin products seemed more and more feasible, I knew that I would build it around high percentages of green tea. Studies had found that green tea is as impressive when applied topically as when taken internally. I knew firsthand, from treating an endless stream of suntanned patients, that we still live in a sun-obsessed world. As a result, I was sure that products rich in antioxidants were sorely needed. Also, many botanicals have been found to have healing and soothing properties, as well as dermatological ingredients like salicylic acid and retinol, both proven to provide tangible improvement in the skin.

Here is the dr. brandt skin care collection.

∶ Overview ∶

The dr. brandt skin care collection is a healthy lifestyle for mind, body, and senses. When it is thought of as a nutritional program for the skin, the daily diet—its basic bread and butter, so to speak—can be found in the core lineless or poreless products.

If your skin is normal, dry, or sensitive, your daily care is in the lineless category. If your skin is combination or oily, you would select a daily diet of products from the poreless category.

When your skin is feeling a little under the weather, the active additives in the dr. brandt skin care products help your skin regain its sparkle.

When you have trouble with your eyes, you see an eye specialist; when you have trouble with your feet, you see a foot specialist. When you have trouble with your skin, you have the specialists, a collection of products for very specific, very special skin care needs. To really get the body back into shape, a physical therapist is your best bet. Similarly, you can rehabilitate your dehabilitated zones with our physical therapy range of products.

dr. brandt skin care is a commitment to the marriage of science and nature. Our custom formulations embrace innovative, world-first technologies created to maintain radiant, glowing skin. dr. brandt skin care formulas are rich with powerful vitamins, shea butter, green tea, grapeseed extract, natural botanicals, blemish-fighting salicylic acid, tea tree, rosemary, and other skin-saving elements. Every product is a dedication to beautiful, younger-looking skin. The difference? These products are formulated under dermatologic control for maximum safety and efficiency and offer the highest performance without a prescription.

dr. brandt skin care

lineless collection

Antioxidant, antiwrinkle, and antiaging prevention and repair are at the heart of dr. brandt's philosophy. The lineless collection merges sky-high percentages of green tea, the antioxidant superpower known for its skin-saving anti-inflammatory properties, with grapeseed extract, renowned for its protecting, firming, and strengthening power. From the deepest cellular level of the skin up to the surface, the lineless collection smooths, protects, repairs, and adds visible radiance to your skin. Recommended as the daily care regimen for normal, dry, or sensitive skins.

lineless gel cleanser: Green tea and conditioners calm and cleanse in one step.

lineless tone for dry/sensitive skin: An antioxidant-rich toner formulated with green tea, chamomile, witch hazel, and soothing botanicals.

lineless cream: Green tea, grapeseed extract, and botanicals provide antiaging benefits in a luxurious cream formula—ideal for normal to dry skin.

lineless gel: Green tea, grapeseed extract, and botanicals provide antiaging benefits in a lightweight gel formula—ideal for combination and oily skin.

lineless eye cream: Rich in soothing and firming vitamins, botanicals, and green tea for a younger-looking eye contour. Exceptional for treating effects of aging, puffiness, and dark circles.

lineless soothing mask: A unique mask with green tea, chamomile, licorice, and aloe to refresh, revive, and renew the complexion.

poreless collection

Formulated for acne-prone skin of all ages, the poreless collection refines enlarged pores, controls excess oil, and balances combination complexions. Anti-irritant and lipid-soluble salicylic acid is paired with antibacterial tea tree to go deep into the pores, dissolving dirt and oils and clearing breakouts. Calming botanicals and zinc oxide reduce the appearance of redness and the uneven skin tone associated with blemished skin. Recommended as the daily care regimen for oily and combination skin types.

poreless cleanser: Formulated with citric extracts and clarifying tea tree and rosemary to dissolve impurities, oils, and debris. Leaves you with that ultraclean sensation.

poreless tone for oily/combination: An invigorating, purifying toner for combination and oily skins.

pore effect: Clarifying cream that combines the power of salicylic acid, antibacterial tea tree, and stimulating rosemary extract. Soothing lavender calms redness and irritations associated with blemished skin. When it is used daily, skin becomes visibly clearer with fewer breakouts. Tightens and refines pores and controls excess oils.

poreless moisture: Balancing, "mattifying," ultrasheer moisture formula for oily and combination skin that will not clog pores and is fragrance-free. Formulated with soothing lavender and toning white birch extract to condition skin.

poreless purifying mask: Formulated with kaolin and bentonite clays and tea tree to deep-clean, draw out impurities, and tighten enlarged pores. Zinc oxide calms redness.

active additives

A few extras that supplement your regimen in a powerful way. Deeply renewing and restorative vitamin-based skin care formulas designed to improve the overall health, firmness, and radiance of your complexion. A unique delivery system, time-released by the skin's natural moisture system, ensures the stability and efficiency of vitamin C. We have harnessed a pure, food-quality vitamin C that perfectly mimics our body's natural ascorbic acid for maximum absorption and firming antioxidant power.

exfoliating facial wash: Geranium- and grapefruit-enriched formula that cleanses and exfoliates in one step. Gentle enough to be used daily.

"c" gel: Cocktail of powerful antioxidants and botanicals that firm, smooth, and fight free radicals, in a potent vitamin C base that stimulates collagen production.

"c" cream: Fight free radicals and firm and hydrate your complexion with this highly potent vitamin C cream.

"c" eye cream: Smooth and firm the total eye area with vitamin C, nourishing shea butter, and soothing chamomile and botanicals.

"a" cream night: Renew, restore, and replenish. Retinol increases cellular turnover while botanicals of green tea and chamomile soothe and protect the skin.

vitamin moisture mask: The name says it all. A perfect blend of vitamins A, C, and E; natural hydrators; and soothing algae extract to instantly beautify and hydrate the skin.

the specialists

These targeted products were developed to meet and exceed your skin care criteria. Using patented technologies developed for advanced results, these products work synergistically with the skin.

anti-irritant cleanser: A mild (nonsoap) creamy cleanser with a soothing action developed for ultrasensitive skin and for those using glycolic acid products.

d-face makeup remover: Whisks away even the most stubborn eye and face makeup without leaving a trace of oil.

v-zone neck cream: Vitamin C and smoothing glycolic acid work together to regenerate and firm the delicate tissue of the neck.

aftershave "c": Unisex postshave formula that firms and conditions using vitamin C, green tea, soothing aloe, and allantoin, the ultimate irritation eradicator.

lightening gel: Fades age spots and hyperpigmentation with a unique formula containing glycolic acid and 2 percent hydroquinone.

infinite moisture for dry/dehydrated skin: Hydrating hyaluronic acid and other soothing botanicals provide extreme hydration and restore elasticity.

Because the skin on your body deserves just as much TLC as the rest of you.

liquid loofah: Buff, soften, and smooth your skin with beads suspended in a foaming gel rich in antioxidants and botanicals.

vitamin "c" body lotion: Regenerating body lotion that firms, soothes, retexturizes, and rehydrates. That special touch: the refreshing sensation of grapefruit extract.

balanced body moisturizer: The ultimate body lotion, formulated with lactic acid to soften dry and chapped skin.

balanced hand cream: Alleviate dry, chapped hands with rich emollient conditioners.

sun

Understanding why the sun is not your friend is only half the battle; having the best sun protection products completes the picture.

spf 15 gel with parsol: A waterproof formula featuring Parsol 1789 for complete UVA and UVB sun protection. Ideal for oily and combination skin, as it will not cause or aggravate breakouts.

spf 15 chemfree: An award-winning sun-shield formula of micronized titanium and zinc oxide (no more white streaks!) and soothing botanicals. The anti-inflammatory superantioxidant green tea provides additional protection from free-radical damage.

spf 30 bronze barrier face (deep): Best under the sun, under the clouds, and under your makeup. Enjoy a sun-kissed look without the sun. This golden-bronze-tinted ultralightweight gel protects your skin from UVA and UVB rays with added antioxidant benefits of green tea and other natural botanicals.

spf 30 bronze barrier face (colorless): Best under the sun, under the clouds, and under your makeup. This colorless ultra-lightweight gel protects your skin from UVA and UVB rays with added antioxidant benefits of green tea and other natural botanicals.

spf 15 body barrier gel, spf 30 body barrier gel: Best under the sun, under the clouds, and all over the body. This colorless ultralightweight gel protects your skin from damaging UVA and UVB rays with the added antioxidant protection of green tea. Geranium and chamomile calms and tones.

dr. brandt skin care products can be found in the following retail outlets:

Select Nordstrom stores, *www.nordstrom.com* and 1-800-7BEAUTY

Sephora, *www.Sephora.com*

Select Neiman Marcus stores

Bergdorf Goodman

Also available at *www.drbrandtskincare.com* and 1-800-234-1066